COVID-19 and Older Adults

This book examines the impact of the pandemic on the older population and how gerontological social workers can effectively intervene to ensure a more equitable approach to service delivery. It details the various ways COVID-19 has touched the lives of older adults and their caregivers across diverse countries including Italy, China, Nigeria, and the United States. Readers of this book can expect comprehensive attention to pandemic issues in an international gerontological social work context.

This edited collection will greatly interest students, academics, and researchers in the humanities and social sciences with an interest in the sociology of aging and the impact of the COVID-19 pandemic. The chapters in this book were originally published as a special issue of *Journal of Gerontological Social Work*.

Robin P. Bonifas is Professor and Chair of the Social Work Department at Indiana State University, Terre Haute, USA. She has over 15 years' experience working with older adults in long-term care and inpatient psychiatric settings. She is John A. Hartford Faculty Scholar and Editor-in-Chief of the *Journal of Gerontological Social Work*.

COVID-19 and Older Adults

Edited by
Robin P. Bonifas

Routledge
Taylor & Francis Group

LONDON AND NEW YORK

First published 2024
by Routledge
4 Park Square, Milton Park, Abingdon, Oxon, OX14 4RN

and by Routledge
605 Third Avenue, New York, NY 10158

Routledge is an imprint of the Taylor & Francis Group, an informa business

© 2024 Taylor & Francis

British Library Cataloguing-in-Publication Data
A catalogue record for this book is available from the British Library

ISBN13: 978-1-032-50903-7 (hbk)
ISBN13: 978-1-032-50907-5 (pbk)
ISBN13: 978-1-003-40027-1 (ebk)

DOI: 10.4324/9781003400271

Typeset in Minion Pro
by codeMantra

Publisher's Note
The publisher accepts responsibility for any inconsistencies that may have arisen during the conversion of this book from journal articles to book chapters, namely the inclusion of journal terminology.

Disclaimer
Every effort has been made to contact copyright holders for their permission to reprint material in this book. The publishers would be grateful to hear from any copyright holder who is not here acknowledged and will undertake to rectify any errors or omissions in future editions of this book.

Contents

Citation Information

The chapters in this book were originally published in the *Journal of Gerontological Social Work*, volume 64, issue 6 (2021). When citing this material, please use the original page numbering for each article, as follows:

For any permission-related enquiries please visit:
http://www.tandfonline.com/page/help/permissions

Notes on Contributors

Patricia Uju Agbawodikeizu, Department of Social Work, University of Nigeria, Nigeria.

Robin P. Bonifas, Social Work Department, Indiana State University, Terre Haute, USA.

Ersilia Brambilla, AUSER Regionale Lombardia, Milan, Italy.

Rino Campioni, AUSER Regionale Lombardia, Milan, Italy.

Wai Chan, Sau Po Centre on Ageing, The University of Hong Kong, Hong Kong.

Johnson Chun Sing Cheung, Department of Social Work and Social Administration, The University of Hong Kong, Hong Kong.

Robert K. Chigangaidze, Faculty of Social Sciences, School of Social Work, Midlands State University, Gweru, Zimbabwe.

Patience Chinyenze, Faculty of Social Sciences, School of Social Work, Midlands State University, Gweru, Zimbabwe.

Cheryl Hiu Kwan Chui, Department of Social Work and Social Administration, The University of Hong Kong, Hong Kong.

Prince Chiagozie Ekoh, Department of Social Work, University of Nigeria, Nigeria.

Chigozie Donatus Ezulike, Department of Social Work, University of Nigeria, Nigeria; Department of Social and Behavioural Sciences, City University of Hong Kong, Kowloon, Hong Kong.

Carla Facchini, Associazione Nestore, Milan, Italy; Department of Sociology and Social Research, Università Degli Studi Di Milano Bicocca, Milan, Italy.

Elizabeth Onyedikachi George, Department of Social Work, University of Nigeria, Nigeria.

Marisa Giorgi, Older Adults Technology Services (OATS), USA.

Alexander Glazebrook, Older Adults Technology Services (OATS), USA.

Erika Guastafierro, UOC Neurology, Public Health, Disability, Fondazione IRCCS Istituto Neurologico Carlo Besta, Milan, Italy.

M. Aaron Guest, Edson College of Nursing and Health Innovation; Center for Innovation in Healthy and Resilient Aging, Arizona State University, Tempe, USA.

Thomas Kamber, Older Adults Technology Services (OATS), USA.

Courtney Kutzler, School of Social Work, University of Minnesota, Minneapolis, USA.

Matilde Leonardi, UOC Neurology, Public Health, Disability, Fondazione IRCCS Istituto Neurologico Carlo Besta, Milan, Italy.

Elizabeth Lightfoot, School of Social Work, University of Minnesota, Minneapolis, USA.

Shiyu Lu, Sau Po Centre on Ageing, The University of Hong Kong, Hong Kong.

Terry Yat Sang Lum, Department of Social Work and Social Administration, The University of Hong Kong, Hong Kong.

Francesca G. Magnani, UOC Neurology, Public Health, Disability, Fondazione IRCCS Istituto Neurologico Carlo Besta, Milan, Italy.

Molly Maxfield, Edson College of Nursing and Health Innovation; Center for Innovation in Healthy and Resilient Aging, Arizona State University, Tempe, USA.

Rajean Moone, Center for Healthy Aging and Innovation, University of Minnesota, Minneapolis, USA.

Ikechukwu Nnebe, Department of Social Work, University of Nigeria, Nigeria.

Uzoma Odera Okoye, Department of Social Work, University of Nigeria, Nigeria.

Jacob Otis, School of Social Work, University of Minnesota, Minneapolis, USA.

Allie Peckham, Edson College of Nursing and Health Innovation; Center for Innovation in Healthy and Resilient Aging, Arizona State University, Tempe, USA.

Keenan A. Pituch, Edson College of Nursing and Health Innovation, Arizona State University, Tempe, USA.

Rosa Romano, AUSER Regionale Lombardia, Milan, Italy.

Kamal Suleiman, Department of Psychology, University of Pennsylvania, Philadelphia, USA.

Claudia Toppo, UOC Neurology, Public Health, Disability, Fondazione IRCCS Istituto Neurologico Carlo Besta, Milan, Italy.

Kenneth Turck, School of Social Work, University of Minnesota, Minneapolis, USA.

Joyce Weil, College of Natural and Health Sciences, University of Northern Colorado, Greeley, USA.

Heejung Yun, School of Social Work, University of Minnesota, Minneapolis, USA.

Kimberly Ziegler, Older Adults Technology Services (OATS), USA.

Introducing *COVID-19 and Older Adults*

Dear Readers,

I am very excited to introduce the first special issue of the *Journal of Gerontological Social Work* focused on COVID-19 and older adults; a second special issue featuring articles addressing this topic will follow later this year. There is so much work being done worldwide to examine the impact of the pandemic on the older population and how gerontological social workers can effectively intervene that it requires two issues to disseminate the research and conceptual frameworks!

This first special issue begins by calling attention to the intersection of ageism and COVID-19. Maxfield and colleagues discuss older adults' fears of receiving stigmatized and biased care due to health provider stereotypes that view them as frail and vulnerable. Chigangaidze and Chinyenze present immunosenescence as a primary risk factor for COVID-19 rather than the aging process itself and encourage a preventative focus that bolsters immune system health among this population as a more equitable approach to service delivery.

This special issue also draws attention to COVID-19-related issues for older adults internationally, with an article examining perception of infection risk in Italy (Guastafierro and colleagues), another investigating associations among post-pandemic volunteering and mental health in China (Chan et al.), and two articles from Nigeria, one assessing the impact of the pandemic on seniors' economic activities and well-being (Agbawodileizu and colleagues), and the other assessing digital exclusion and social isolation (Ekoh et al.).

Using a U.S. sample, Weil et al. also focus on digital exclusion of older people and help reframe the relationship of older adults to technology such that it can be viewed in a positive light for greater digital inclusion. Employing a similar positive focus, Lightfoot et al. present interview findings from older adult caregivers, which reveal both the special joys and the challenges of caregiving during the pandemic.

This special issue ends with a book review of Doka and Tucci's *Living with Grief since COVID-19* by Anderson, which highlights the personal narratives of the grief from diverse individuals impacted by the virus.

As always, I hope you enjoy reading the informative articles in this issue.

Disclosure statement

No potential conflict of interest was reported by the author(s).

Robin P. Bonifas

Age-Based Healthcare Stereotype Threat during the COVID-19 Pandemic

Molly Maxfield ⓘD, Allie Peckham ⓘD, M. Aaron Guest ⓘD
and Keenan A. Pituch ⓘD

ABSTRACT
Older adults have been identified as a high-risk population for COVID-19 by the United States Centers for Disease Control and Prevention (CDC). Though well-intentioned, this nonspecific designation highlights stereotypes of older adults as frail and in need of protection, exacerbating negative age-based stereotypes that can have adverse effects on older adults' well-being. Healthcare stereotype threat (HCST) is concern about being judged by providers and receiving biased medical treatment based on stereotypes about one's identity – in this case age. Given the attention to older adults' physical vulnerabilities during the COVID-19 pandemic, older adults may be especially worried about age-based judgments from medical providers and sensitive to ageist attitudes about COVID-19. Online data collection (April 13 to May 15, 2020) with adults aged 50 and older ($N = 2325$, $M = 63.11$, $SD = 7.53$) examined age-based HCST. Respondents who worried that healthcare providers judged them based on age ($n = 584$) also reported more negative COVID-19 reactions, including perceived indifference toward older adults, young adults' lack of concern about health, and unfavorable media coverage of older adults. The results highlight the intersection of two pandemics: COVID-19 and ageism. We close with consideration of the clinical implications of the results.

The COVID-19 pandemic has been disruptive for individuals of all ages. However, older adults are considered a high-risk group based on higher mortality rates and significant long-term effects of COVID-19. This designation is at least partially due to older adults' higher rates of preexisting comorbidities (e.g., cardiovascular disease, hypertension, diabetes, chronic respiratory disease, and chronic kidney disease) that have been associated with more severe COVID-19 outcomes (Shahid et al., 2020). Perhaps for these reasons, public officials in the United States have recommended that older adults take extreme precautions, including isolation, without consistently providing a more specific range of ages at risk (for commentary, see Berridge & Hooyman, 2020). Certainly, a disproportionate number of COVID-19 related deaths in the United States occur in adults aged 65 and older (8 in 10 by some estimates), and risk of hospitalization and death increase by decade (18–29 year olds as comparison), with greatest risks among individuals aged 85 and older (CDC, 2020). However, vague designations of older adults and age-related COVID-19 risks do not account for the diversity in health status within older adults (Fingerman & Trevino, 2020) and perpetuate the use of oversimplified age-based judgments, also known as stereotypes (Ayalon et al., 2020).

Stereotypes about older adults are predominantly negative (Kite et al., 2005) and often focus on physical and cognitive decline (e.g., frail, slow, forgetful, dependent, etc.). Palmore (2004) found that among older adults from both Canada and the United States, almost half reported that a doctor or nurse attributed their medical problem to their age. Older adults themselves may attribute health problems to their age, which contributes to avoidance of healthcare services (Goodwin et al., 1999). The frequency of age-related attributions for health status raises concerns about the role of stereotypes and stereotype threat in healthcare. Stereotype threat is the concern about being reduced to and/or affirming negative stereotypes associated with one's identity (e.g., Steele et al., 2002). Originally investigated with young adults, known negative consequences of stereotype threat, such as elevated blood pressure (e.g., Blascovich et al., 2001) and reduced working memory (e.g., Schmader & Johns, 2003) have clear relevance for older adults. In experimental studies including older adults, activation of age-related stereotypes contributes to poorer cognitive and physical functioning compared to control conditions (for a review, see Barber, 2020).

Healthcare stereotype threat (HCST) focuses on concerns about being reduced to or reinforcing stereotypes about one's group, specifically those relevant to healthcare settings and health-related behavior (Abdou et al., 2016). HCST is believed to contribute to health disparities; individuals who worry healthcare providers judge them based on race/ethnicity, gender, age, weight, socioeconomic status, or other reasons (or combination of stereotypes) also report poorer self-perceived health and are more likely to have hypertension and depressive symptoms compared to respondents who do not report HCST (Abdou et al., 2016). The combination of two or more types of HCST (perceived judgments based on weight *and* race, for example) increase the likelihood for all three of those outcomes (Abdou et al., 2016). Additionally, HCST predicts greater distrust of the provider and lower perceived quality of care (Abdou et al., 2016), which may result in avoidance of healthcare altogether (Aaronson et al., 2013). Though the specific mechanism leading to stereotype threat and HCST effects is unclear, one potential explanation related to stereotype threat is the tendency to avoid stereotype-relevant domains (Steele et al., 2002). For example, patients worried about being judged about their age may avoid situations in which age could be a focus, such as a healthcare appointment. Of additional concern, if stereotype threat in a healthcare setting leads to physiological arousal and reduced working memory, patients may be less able to attend to, and later recall, important information conveyed during appointments. For these reasons alone, it can be helpful to engage in team-based care to facilitate patient understanding and appropriate follow-up care (Schottenfeld et al., 2016), including follow-up appointments to ensure patients are following recommendations.

Heightened attention to age and older adults' vulnerability (accurate or not) during the COVID-19 pandemic raises concerns about age-based HCST. Age-related stereotypes and judgments during the pandemic are particularly visible and include media narratives appearing to reflect an attitude of "disposability" of older adults (Lichtenstein, 2020). Among young adults, hostile ageism predicted lower prioritization of COVID-19 testing, intensive treatment, and vaccination for older adults (Apriceno et al., 2021). Similar age-based judgments regarding healthcare priorities are reflected in calls to ration care to older individuals (Miller, 2020). Media coverage equating age with vulnerability, unclear public health messages about age within the United States, and emphasis on the costs of caring for older adults all align with existing negative age stereotypes and may raise older adults' concern about being reduced to a stereotype (particularly in healthcare settings) and worries about COVID-19 in general. Awareness of the extent to which individuals aged 50 and older experience HCST may spark providers' awareness of overreliance on age as a clinical indicator and its impact on patients and clients. Given the many uncertainties of the effects of COVID-19, clinical social workers are particularly well positioned to be a vital part of integrated behavioral health teams and promote understanding of factors influencing health and health-seeking behaviors.

Present study

Widespread media coverage in the United States has labeled COVID-19 as a health problem for older adults, emphasizing existing age-related stereotypes of physical vulnerability. We thus anticipated high rates of age-based HCST among adults aged 50 and older, relative to similar questions asked of adults aged 50 and older prior to the pandemic (Abdou et al., 2016; Phibbs & Hooker, 2018). Since initiating this study, an investigation of HCST in Israel (March 29 to May 3, 2020; Cohn-Schwartz & Ayalon, 2020) has been published, providing an opportunity for comparison of HCST between Israel and United States. We also predicted that reports of age-based HCST during an age-focused pandemic, in which United States' public health messages were broad and shifting, would be associated with greater concerns about COVID-19 in general.

Method

Participants

Adults aged 50 and older were invited to participate in an online survey (Harris et al., 2009) about COVID-19. Although 2325 started the study, 1705 responded to all items included in the analyses. The treatment of missing data is described in the Statistical Analysis section below.

Procedure

Procedures were approved by the Institutional Review Board. An online survey concerning COVID-19 was advertised on list-serves, university forums, and social media. Interested individuals could provide their e-mail address for entry in a lottery for one of three 20 USD gift cards. The findings reported here represent a small portion of a larger study designed to assess the COVID-19 pandemic's impact on health, healthcare access, well-being, and social support; completing the entire survey took approximately 15 to 25 minutes. Data collection occurred April 13 to May 15, 2020. We describe only those variables included in analyses.

Measures

After providing informed consent, participants were asked to report basic demographic information. They also provided single-item ratings of self-perceived health (1 = *very bad* to 5 = *very good*) and self-perceived risk for COVID-19 (1 = *not risk at all* to 5 = *very high risk*).

Chronic health conditions
Participants indicated on a checklist whether they had been diagnosed with common chronic health conditions, such as high blood pressure and kidney disease, among others (CDC, 2019). Positive responses were summed, with higher numbers indicating a greater number of chronic conditions. Sum scores could range from zero to 21 (actual responses ranged from zero to 12). This checklist and the aforementioned rating of self-perceived health were included as participants in poorer objective or subjective health may also perceive the pandemic differently.

Age-based healthcare stereotype threat

The age-based HCST assessment was based on a question from the Health and Retirement Study (HRS; 2012 wave, Module 8) used in similar studies (e.g., Abdou et al., 2016; Phibbs & Hooker, 2018). We modified the question slightly to focus on judgments based on age only (whereas the HRS assessed age, race, gender, weight, etc.) and to inquire more generally about healthcare providers rather than "doctor or other medical staff." Specifically, participants in the present study were asked: "When you go for medical appointments, do you worry that healthcare providers make judgments about you because of your age?" As in the HRS, response options included yes, no, or I don't know.

COVID-19 reactions

Next, participants indicated reactions to the COVID-19 pandemic, including general questions about testing availability and age-related questions concerning perceived indifference about older adults contracting the virus. Participants indicate agreement with each statement on a scale of 1 (*strongly disagree*) to 5 (*strongly agree*). This measure was created for the present study shortly after the United States declared the COVID-19 outbreak a national emergency (March, 2020); it is briefly described along with the exploratory factor analysis conducted to identify underlying constructs. Mean scores were calculated for each subscale. Scale items are available in the supplemental material.

Statistical analysis

We first examined basic descriptive statistics, frequencies, and various plots to identify if implausible values were present, determine the extent of incomplete data, and screen for possible violations of assumptions. Note that although data were incomplete, we used appropriate missing data treatments, as described below. We also examined index plots (e.g., Mahalanobis' distance and various influence measures) to assess if multivariate outliers and influential observations were present. Such observations were present for some analyses, but inclusion or exclusion of these cases did not alter any study conclusions.

Three different analyses were used to address our research questions. First, to obtain and test for differences in the proportions of participants in the HCST categories, we used multinomial logistic regression and estimated parameters with maximum likelihood estimation (MLE). Second, given that we created a measure of participant reactions to the COVID-19 pandemic, including general and age-related questions, we conducted exploratory factor analysis (EFA) to identify underlying constructs. We estimated EFA models with the number of factors varying from one to four with the oblique geomin rotation method used. Following recommendations in Pituch and Stevens

(2016), we defined a well-fitting model as one where the comparative fit (CFI) and Tucker-Lewis indices (TLI) each exceed a value of .90, and the root mean square error of approximation (RMSEA) and the standardized root mean square residual (SRMR) are each less than .05. For the EFA, parameters were estimated by a maximum likelihood procedure (i.e., MLR) that is robust to violations of normality and provides for optimal parameter estimates when data are missing at random (Enders & Bandalos, 2001; Savalei, 2010). Note that for the analyses described above, MLE removes cases that provide no data on any of the outcome variables. As such, some cases were removed automatically by the procedure because they make no contribution to parameter estimation. Although in principle, auxiliary variables could be included to potentially improve missing data treatment, no study variable was correlated with any outcome at a value of |.40| or greater, which is recommended for inclusion of auxiliary variables (Enders, 2010).

Third, to assess the degree to which study predictors were related to the resultant EFA factors, we used exploratory structural equation modeling, or ESEM (Asparouhov & Muthén, 2009). Estimating a model that includes all EFA derived factors and corresponding items whose loading exceeded a value of |.30|, we regressed the set of factors on the study predictors. The advantages of using ESEM are that it uses (a) the factors obtained from the EFA analysis without needing to compute factor scores or composite variables and (b) MLE to treat incomplete data at the item-level. In addition to the outcome variables, we applied MLE missing data treatment to incomplete predictors such that information from all cases in the study were used to estimate model parameters. Mplus software, version 8.5 (Muthén & Muthén, 1998–2020) was used to implement the primary analyses. We used the default z tests to assess the significance of parameter estimates, with alpha set to 0.05. To test interactions between age and HCST, we used the omnibus multivariate Wald test, which if significant, was followed-up with z tests that assessed the association between age and a given outcome for each HCST group, as well as z tests that assessed if such associations differed across these groups.

Results

See Table 1 for participant characteristics by HCST response.

Age-based healthcare stereotype threat

The multinomial logistic regression indicated that almost a third of participants who responded to this item (n = 584, 31.1%) reported worry about age-based judgments from healthcare providers, a majority does not worry (n = 1108, 59.0%), and 10% of participants reported that

Table 1. Participant characteristics by response to HCST.

Variable	Yes n = 584		No n = 1108		I don't know n = 186	
	M	SD	M	SD	M	SD
Age	63.91	7.34	62.76	7.60	62.77	7.59
Per Health	4.05	.79	4.21	.73	4.03	.78
CHC Sum	2.58	2.02	2.44	1.83	2.35	1.86
Per COVID-19 risk	3.18	1.01	3.01	1.00	3.03	.98
Indifference toward OA	3.36	.93	2.84	.90	3.27	.80
YA unconcerned	3.98	1.00	3.83	1.01	4.04	.90
COVID-19 worry	4.03	.79	3.93	.77	3.92	.79
Unfavorable media	3.61	1.08	3.10	1.07	3.38	.96
	n	%	n	%	n	%
Gender						
Women	526	90.1	942	85.0	161	86.6
Men	56	9.6	163	14.7	25	13.4
Missing	2	0.3	3	0.3	0	0.0
Ethnicity						
Non-Hispanic	457	78.3	851	76.8	137	73.7
Hispanic	20	3.4	27	2.4	2	1.1
Missing	107	18.3	230	20.8	47	25.3
Race						
White	457	78.3	842	76.0	132	71.0
Black/African American	3	0.5	4	0.4	2	1.1
Asian	1	0.2	4	0.4	1	0.5
Pacific Islander	1	0.2	0	0.0	0	0.0
Other	13	2.2	14	1.3	2	1.1
Multiracial	4	0.7	6	0.5	3	1.6
Missing	105	18.0	238	21.5	46	24.7
Country of Residence						
US†	457	78.3	849	76.6	131	70.4
Other	22	3.8	31	2.8	10	5.4
Missing	105	18.0	228	20.6	45	24.2

Note: † = a greater proportion than reported are presumed to be residents of the United States, as the study was largely advertised locally and nationally; however, missing data for this item prevent us from confirming this.
HCST = healthcare stereotype threat (worry about health care providers' judgments based on your age). OA = older adult. YA = young adult. Per Health = self-perceived health (1 = *very bad* to 5 = *very good*), CHC Sum = sum of chronic health conditions indicated (possible range = 0-21), Per COVID-19 risk = self-perceived COVID-19 risk (1 = *no risk at all* to 5 = *very high risk*).

they do not know ($n = 186$, 9.9%). Pairwise comparisons among the categories indicated that statistically significant differences were present between each category and the others (each p-value < .001). Four hundred forty-seven participants did not respond to this item.

Exploratory factor analysis

Of the factor models fit to the data, only the four factor model met each of the characteristics of a good-fitting model, with CFI = .99, TLI = .98, RMSEA = .03 and SRMR = .01. We labeled the resultant factors "perceived indifference toward older adults" (3 items; α = .76), "young adults less concerned about health" (2 items; α = .85), "COVID-19 worry" (4 items; α = .68), and "unfavorable media portrayal of older adults" (2 items; α = .90). One item did not load on any of the factors and was removed from the analysis. See supplemental material for scale items, factor loadings, and factor correlations, which vary in magnitude and are all positive as expected.

Responses to COVID-19

Table 2 shows the ESEM regression results prior to including age-by-HCST interactions. The models for each factor were significant: indifference toward older adults, $R^2 = .23$, $z = 10.95$, $p < .001$, young adults less concerned about health, $R^2 = .09$, $z = 6.54$, $p < .001$, COVID-19 worry, $R^2 = .23$, $z = 10.68$, $p < .001$, and unfavorable media portrayal of older adults, $R^2 = .09$, $z = 6.78$, $p < .001$. Greater perceived indifference toward older adults was endorsed by younger and female participants, as well as those who reported poorer perceived health, a greater number of health conditions, greater perceived personal COVID-19 risk, and indicated "yes" or "do not know" to experiencing HCST. Higher scores for the factor "young adults less concerned about health" were obtained by participants indicating fewer health conditions, greater perceived personal COVID-19 risk, and "yes" or "do not know" to experiencing HCST. Greater COVID-19 worry was indicated by females and participants reporting a greater number of health conditions and greater perceived personal COVID-19 risk. Finally, less favorable media

Table 2. Regression Results for Predictors of COVID-19 Reactions.

Variable	Indifference Toward Older Adults			Young Adults Less Concerned About Health			COVID-19 Worry			Unfavorable Media Portrayal of Older Adults		
	B	SE	β	B	SE	β	B	SE	β	B	SE	β
Age	−.01	<.01	−.07*	<.01	< .01	.01	.01	<.01	.04	.01	<.01	.08*
Gender	−.24	.08	−.21*	−.10	.07	−.09	−.48	.09	−.42**	−.45	.08	−.43*
Per Health	−.13	.04	−.09*	<.01	.04	<.01	.04	.04	.02	.06	.04	.05
CHC Sum	.04	.02	.06†	.05	.02	.09*	.04	.02	.07†	−.02	.02	−.04
Per COVID-19 risk	.31	.03	.28**	.26	.03	.25**	.49	.03	.44**	.12	.03	.11**
HCST												
"Yes" vs." no"	.68	.06	.60**	.13	.05	.13†	−.02	.06	−.01	.49	.06	.46**
"Don't know" vs." no"	.58	.10	.51**	.24	.08	.23*	−.07	.10	−.06	.28	.09	.27*
"Yes" vs. "don't know"	.10	.10	.09	−.11	.09	−.11	.05	.10	.05	.20	.09	.20†
R^2	.23**			.09**			.23**			.09**		

Note: † < .05, * ≤ .01, ** ≤ .001

Gender (0 = female, 1 = male); Per Health = self-perceived health (1 = *very bad* to 5 = *very good*), CHC Sum = sum of chronic health conditions indicated, Per COVID-19 risk = self-perceived COVID-19 risk (1 = *no risk at all* to 5 = *very high risk*); HCST = healthcare stereotype threat (worry about healthcare providers' judgments based on your age, a trichotomous variable, with yes, no, and don't know categories). Standardized coefficients for dichotomous predictors (i.e., gender, HCST) were calculated as β = B/SDy, where SDy is the standard deviation of a given outcome variable.

portrayals of older adults was endorsed by older and female participants, those who indicated higher personal COVID-19 risk, and participants who indicated "yes" or "do not know" to experiencing HCST, with those responding "yes" to HCST reporting the most unfavorable media portrayals among the HCST groups.[1]

Discussion

Almost a third of adults aged 50 and older reported worry about being judged by a healthcare provider because of their age; the present proportion (M_{age} = 63.11; 31.1%) was surprisingly high compared to rates reported with another sample of adults aged 50 and older in the United States before the COVID-19 pandemic (M_{age} = 65.9; 8.3% in Abdou et al., 2016). HCST rates were closer to, yet still higher, than those among Israeli adults aged 50 and older during the pandemic (M_{age} = 63.24; 23.65% in Cohn-Schwartz & Ayalon, 2020). Frequency of worry about age-based judgments in the present study is significant within the context of the ongoing COVID-19 pandemic and ongoing media coverage of which often depicts older adults as a "problem" (e.g., Lichtenstein, 2020). Of importance, if age-based HCST is associated with some of the same consequences observed in stereotype threat studies with young adults (e.g., increased anxiety and blood pressure, reduced working memory and self-control), it could have negative and significant influence on older adults' health. Although more specific studies are needed to establish effects of age-based HCST, there is some indication that negative age-stereo-types lead to adverse outcomes relevant to health. For example, after reading portrayals of negative aging stereotypes, older adult participants reported more loneliness and poorer subjective health compared to those who read positive or neutral portrayals (Coudin & Alexopoulos, 2010).

Additionally, individuals experiencing age-based HCST and individuals who were uncertain of whether they were being judged by providers based on their age also expressed greater perceived indifference toward older adults, along with greater perception of the young being less concerned with health and greater perception of unfavorable media portrayal of older adults. That responses of individuals who were unsure about the experience of HCST were so similar to individuals who did report HCST was unexpected, but appears to highlight the power of age-based judgments. Only those who denied concern about age-based judgments from providers reported lower COVID-19 reactions.

That experiencing HCST was associated with greater perception of indif-ference toward older adults' health, young adults being less concerned with health, and unfavorable media attention is perhaps predictable; all three out-comes reflect a form of ageism, be it lack of regard for older adults' health or accurate and thoughtful portrayals of older adults in the media. The single data collection point prevents establishing causal order, leaving it unclear whether people who perceived greater indifference toward older adults and insensitive media portrayals are more sensitive to age-based HCST or vice versa. It would be important to determine whether perceived indifference toward older adults' health and HCST contribute to avoidance of medical appointments, as previous research has suggested that stereotype threat contributes to avoidance of situations in which the stereotype may be activated (Aaronson et al., 2013; Steele et al., 2002).

Study limitations

The homogeneity of the convenience sample is a significant limitation. The predominantly female and White sample is not representative of the population and prevents generalizability of the findings; however, it is reasonable to anticipate that a more racially and ethnically diverse sample would report even greater worry about judgments in health care, though they may attribute them to multiple aspects of their identity. The intersection of age with race and ethnicity in HCST is an important area for future research because the odds for negative outcomes (e.g., poorer self-rated health, hypertension, and depressive symptoms) increase as individuals perceive HCST based on multiple components of their identity (Abdou et al., 2016), in addition to the disproportionately high rates of COVID-19 mortality for Hispanic and Black individuals (Gross et al., 2020). Another study limitation is the single time point collection occurring after COVID-19 was declared a pandemic, which prevents a determination of whether perceived age-based judgments have increased since COVID-19's onset. However, HRS data from 2012 used similar questions and revealed only 8.3% of adults aged 50 and older worried about age-based judgments by a healthcare provider (Abdou et al., 2016). Although not a direct comparison, the present data suggest concerns about age-based judgments are now more prevalent. As noted above, the single time point of data collection also prevents determination of whether perceived HCST led to greater reactions to COVID-19 or vice versa. Additionally, the Reactions to the COVID-19 Pandemic Scale was created soon after the national emergency was declared, so associated psychometric data are limited. Finally, the sample was quite healthy; only 51 people perceived their health as "very bad" or bad" and 1754 rated their health as "very good" or "good," in spite of the fact that 78.5% had one or more chronic health conditions. With a less healthy sample, HCST and COVID-19 worries may be even higher.

Implications for social work practice

Social workers have been a critical conduit of information and resources for older adults during the COVID-19 pandemic. In many ways, traditional social work practice has been upended through the sudden movement to telehealth, a medium that may leave some older adults feeling excluded (Seifert, 2020).

The current results reveal an additional concern working with older adults during the pandemic: that they may be less likely to reach out to seek help due to (mis)perceptions about their age. Social workers should continue to advocate for patient outreach and engagement, particularly encouraging older adults to seek needed services.

There are some promising methods for reducing stereotype threat's impact. Though a detailed review is outside this article's scope, Spencer et al. (2016) review three basic intervention approaches. Reconstrual often involves altering the presentation or the information to minimize or eliminate references to the stereotyped group or stereotypical traits. In the present moment, reconstrual could involve talking with older adults about COVID-19 within the context of multiple factors (e.g., the combination of current health status, risk for exposure, and access to healthcare when needed) rather than focusing only on age. Coping approaches may use self-affirmations to diminish the impact of a stereotype on one's view of self. Here, using a positive frame to highlight the resources older adults do have to manage their health and well-being may reduce effects of stereotypes (as seen on cognitive tasks in Barber et al., 2019). Finally, creating identity safe environments may reduce the presence and impact of stereotype threat. This approach may mean working within one's organizations to ensure age-appropriate and age-friendly marketing of services to best support older adult participation. The Reframing Aging Guidelines offer suggestions for effective and inclusive communication strategies and can be accessed online (Institute, 2017).

Conclusions

The findings reveal a substantial proportion of adults aged 50 and older experience age-based HCST. Further, among individuals who endorse age-based HCST and those who are unsure of whether they are being judged based on their age also report greater perceived indifference toward older adults, less concern about health among youth, and more unfavorable portrayal of older adults in the media. The ageist tone of COVID-19 coverage likely contributes to age discrimination, negative age stereotypes, and negative perceptions about aging within older adults themselves – one manifestation of this appears to be high rates of worry about age-related HCST. Age is undeniably associated with negative outcomes from COVID-19, yet reliance on chronological age is not only an oversimplified way of determining risks for a large, heterogeneous portion of the population, but also contributes to enduring negative stereotypes of older adults. Compounding the problem, the recommendation that older adults socially distance during the pandemic creates an additional threat to physical and psychological health via increased risk for loneliness and social isolation (for a review, see NASEM, 2020). Encouragingly, recent findings suggest that more positive perceptions of aging are protective from distress and loneliness among older adults during COVID-19 related lockdown (Losada-Baltar et al., 2020), and for longer-term solutions, ageist attitudes are generally responsive to intervention (for a review, see Burnes et al., 2019). Ageism adds billions to already high healthcare costs (Levy et al., 2020), providing further incentive to address ageism and associated stereotypes during a pandemic characterized by age-based discrimination and stereotyping.

Note

1. Given the wide age range of participants in the present study, age by HCST interactions were examined in the reported regression model; one interaction was significant. Though not the focus of the article, interested readers may review the results associated with the age by gender interaction in supplemental material. We also included age by gender interactions in the regression model; no such interactions were present for any outcome ($ps > .43$)

Disclosure

We have no known conflicts of interest to disclose.

ORCID

Molly Maxfield (iD) http://orcid.org/0000-0002-3502-2176
Allie Peckham (iD) http://orcid.org/0000-0001-6199-6903
M. Aaron Guest (iD) http://orcid.org/0000-0001-7356-3734
Keenan A. Pituch (iD) http://orcid.org/0000-0003-0768-6490

References

Aaronson, J., Burgess, D., Phelan, S. M., & Jaurez, L. (2013). Unhealthy interactions: The role of stereotype threat in health disparities. *American Journal of Public Health*, *103*(1), 50–56. https://doi.org/10.2105/AJPH.2012.300828

Abdou, C. M., Fingerhut, A. W., Jackson, J. S., & Wheaton, F. (2016). Healthcare stereotype threat in older adults in the Health and Retirement Study. *American Journal of Preventative Medicine*, *50*(2), 191–198. http://dx.doi.org/10.1016/j.amepre.2015.07.034

Apriceno, M., Lytle, A., Monahan, C., Macdonald, J., & Levy, S. R. (2021). Prioritizing health care and employment resources during COVID-19: Roles of benevolent and hostile ageism. *The Gerontologist*, *61*(1), 98–102. https://doi.org/10.1093/geront/gnaa165

Asparouhov, T., & Muthén, B. (2009). Exploratory structural equation modeling. *Structural Equation Modeling: A Multidisciplinary Journal*, *16*(3), 397–438. https://doi.org/10.1080/10705510903008204

Ayalon, L., Chasteen, A., Diehl, M., Levy, B., Neupert, S. D., Rothermund, K., Tesch-Römer, C., & Wahl, H.-W. (2020). Aging in times of the COVID-19 pandemic: Avoiding ageism and fostering intergenerational solidarity. *Journals of Gerontology, Series B: Psychological Sciences and Social Sciences, 76*(2), e49-e52. https://doi.org/10.1093/geronb/gbaa051

Barber, S. J. (2020). The applied implications of age-based stereotype threat for older adults. *Journal of Applied Research in Memory and Cognition, 9*(3), 274–285. https://doi.org/10.1016/j.jarmac.2020.05.002

Barber, S. J., Seliger, J., Yeh, N., & Tan, S. C. (2019). Stereotype threat reduces the positivity of older adults' recall. *Journals of Gerontology Series B: Psychological Sciences and Social Sciences, 74*(4), 585–594. https://doi.org/10.1093/geronb/gby026

Berridge, C., & Hooyman, N. (2020). The consequences of ageist language are upon us. *Journal of Gerontological Social Work, 63*(6–7), 508–512. https://doi.org/10.1080/01634372.2020.1764688

Blascovich, J., Spencer, S. J., Quinn, D., & Steele, C. (2001). African Americans and high blood pressure: The role of stereotype threat. *Psychological Science, 12*(3), 225–229. https://doi.org/10.1111/1467-9280.00340

Burnes, D., Sheppard, C., Henderson, C. R., Wassel, M., Cope, R., Barber, C., & Pillemer, K. (2019). Interventions to reduce ageism against older adults: A systematic review and meta-analysis. *American Journal of Public Health, 109*(8), E1–E9. https://doi.org/10.2105/AJPH.2019.305123

CDC. (2019). *Behavioral risk factor surveillance system questionnaire.* https://www.cdc.gov/brfss/questionnaires/pdf-ques/2017_BRFSS_Pub_Ques_508_tagged.pdf

CDC. (2020). *Older adults at greater risk of requiring hospitalization or dying if diagnosed with COVID-19.* Retrieved January 14, 2021, from https://www.cdc.gov/coronavirus/2019-ncov/need-extra-precautions/older-adults.html

Cohn-Schwartz, E., Ayalon, L., & Carr, D. S. (2020). Societal views of older adults as vulnerable and a Burden to society during the COVID-19 outbreak: results from an Israeli nationally representative sample. *The Journals of Gerontology: Series B.* https://doi.org/10.1093/geronb/gbaa150

Coudin, G., & Alexopoulos, T. (2010). 'Help me! I'm old!' How negative aging stereotypes create dependency among older adults. *Aging & Mental Health, 14*(5), 516–523. https://doi.org/10.1080/13607861003713182

Enders, C. K. (2010). *Applied missing data analysis.* Guilford Press.

Enders, C. K., & Bandalos, D. L. (2001). The relative performance of full information maximum likelihood estimation for missing data in structural equation models. *Structural Equation Modeling, 8*(3), 430–457. https://doi.org/10.1207/S15328007SEM0803_5

Fingerman, K. L., & Trevino, K. (2020, April 7). *Don't lump seniors together on coronavirus. Older people aren't all the same. USA Today.* https://www.usatoday.com/story/opinion/2020/04/07/coronavirus-seniors-lead-diverse-lives-death-rate-varies-column/2954897001/

Goodwin, J. S., Black, S. A., & Satish, S. (1999). Aging versus disease: The opinions of older Black, Hispanic, and non-Hispanic White Americans about the causes and treatment of common medical conditions. *Journal of the American Geriatrics Society, 47*(8), 973–979. https://doi.org/10.1111/j.1532-5415.1999.tb01293.x

Gross, C. P., Essien, U. R., Pasha, S., Gross, J. R., Wang, S., & Nunez-Smith, M. (2020). Racial and ethnic disparities in population level COVID-19 mortality. *Journal of General Internal Medicine, 35*(10), 3097–3099. https://doi.org/10.1007/s11606-020-06081-w

Harris, P. A., Taylor, R., Thielke, R., Payne, J., Gonzalez, N., & Conde, J. G. (2009). Research electronic data capture (REDCap)—A metadata-driven methodology and workflow process for providing translational research informatics support. *Journal of Biomedical Informatics, 42*(2), 377–381. https://doi.org/10.1016/j.jbi.2008.08.010

Institute, F. (2017). *Framing strategies to advance aging and address ageism as policy issues.* Frame Brief, Issue.

Kite, M. E., Stockdale, G. D., Whitley, B. E., Jr., & Johnson, B. T. (2005). Attitudes toward younger and older adults: An updated meta-analytic review. *Journal of Social Issues, 61*(2), 241–266. https://doi.org/10.1111/j.1540-4560.2005.00404.x

Levy, B. R., Slade, M. D., Change, E.-S., Kannoth, S., & Wang, S. Y. (2020). Ageism amplifies cost and prevalence of health conditions. *The Gerontologist, 60*(1), 174–181. https://doi.org/10.1093/geront/gny131

Lichtenstein, B. (2020). From "coffin dodger" to "boomer remover": Outbreaks of ageism in three countries with divergent approaches to coronavirus control. *The Journals of Gerontology. Series B, Psychological Sciences and Social Sciences, 76*(4), e206-e212. https://doi.org/10.1093/geronb/gbaa102

Losada-Baltar, A., Jiménez-Gonzalo, L., Gallego-Alberto, L., Del-sequeros Pedroso-chaparro, M., Fernandes-Pires, J., & Márquez-González, M. (2020). "We are staying at home." Association of self-perceptions of aging, personal and family resources, and loneliness with psychological distress during the lock-down period of COVID-19. *The Journals of Gerontology: Series B, Psychological Sciences and Social Sciences, 76*(2), e10e-16. https://doi.10.1093/geronb/gbaa048

Miller, F. G. (2020, April 9). *Why I support age-related rationing of ventilators for Covid-19 patients. The Hastings Center.* https://www.thehastingscenter.org/why-i-support-age-related-rationing-of-ventilators-for-covid-19-patients/

Muthén, L. K., & Muthén, B. O. (1998–2020). *Mplus user's guide* (8th ed.). Muthén & Muthén.

National Academies of Sciences, Engineering, & Medicine. (2020). *Social isolation and loneliness in older adults: Opportunities for the health care system.* The National Academies Press. https://doi.10.17226/25663

Palmore, E. B. (2004). Research note: Ageism in Canada and the United States. *Journal of Cross-Cultural Gerontology, 19*(1), 41–46. https://doi.org/10.1023/B:JCCG.0000015098.62691.ab

Phibbs, S., & Hooker, K. (2018). An exploration of factors associated with ageist stereotype threat in a medical setting. *The Journals of Gerontology. Series B, Psychological Sciences and Social Sciences, 73*(7), 1160–1165. https://doi.org/10.1093/geronb/gbx034

Pituch, K. A., & Stevens, J. P. (2016). *Applied multivariate statistics for the social sciences: Analyses using SAS and IBM's SPSS* (6th ed.). Routledge.

Savalei, V. (2010). Expected versus observed information in SEM with incomplete normal and nonnormal data. *Psychological Methods, 15*(4), 352–367. https://doi.org/10.1037/a0020143

Schmader, T., & Johns, M. (2003). Converging evidence that stereotype threat reduces working memory capacity. *Journal of Social and Personality Psychology, 85*(3), 440–452. https://doi.org/10.1037/0022-3514.85.3.440

Schottenfeld, L., Petersen, D., Peikes, D., Ricciardi, R., Burak, H., McNellis, R., & Genevro, J. (2016). *Creating patient-centered team-based primary care.* AHRQ Pub. No. 16-0002-EF. Agency for Healthcare Research and Quality.

Seifert, A. (2020). The digital exclusion of older adults during the COVID-19 pandemic. *Journal of Gerontological Social Work, 63*(6-7), 674-696. https://doi.org/10.1080/01634372.2020.1764687

Shahid, Z., Kalayanamitra, R., McClafferty, B., Kepko, D., Ramgobin, D., Patel, R., Aggarwal, C. S., Vunnman, R., Sahu, N., Bhatt, D., Jones, K., Golarmari, R., & Jain, R. (2020). COVID-19 and older adults: What we know. *Journal of the American Geriatrics Society, 68*(5), 926–929. https://doi.org/10.1111/jgs.16472

Spencer, S.J., Logel, C., & Davies, P.G. (2016). Stereotype threat. *Annual Review of Psychology, 67*(1), 415–437. doi: 10.1146/annurev-psych-073115-103235.

Steele, C. M., Spencer, S. J., & Aronson, J. (2002). Contending with group image: The psychology of stereotype and social identity threat. *Advances in Experimental Social Psychology, 34*, 379–440. http://dx.doi.org/10.1016S0065-2601(02)80009-0

Older Adults' Risk Perception during the COVID-19 Pandemic in Lombardy Region of Italy: A Cross-sectional Survey

Erika Guastafierro, Claudia Toppo ⓘD, Francesca G. Magnani, Rosa Romano, Carla Facchini, Rino Campioni, Ersilia Brambilla and Matilde Leonardi

ABSTRACT

During COVID-19 pandemic, older adults are the segment of the population at higher health risk. Given the important role the risk perception has in influencing both the behaviors and psychological well-being, it appears useful exploring this factor in this segment of the population. Despite different studies already described the factors influencing the risk perception, few focused on older adults. For this reason, we investigated risk perception in 514 people over 60 years during the lockdown. We administered a structured interview collecting socio-demographic information, sources of information used, actions undertaken to avoid contagion, and risk perception. Risk perception related to COVID-19 was significantly lower than the perceived risk associated with other threats, and it was correlated to the number of sources of information used but not to the actions undertaken. Furthermore, we found higher risk perception in who knew infected persons, and a negative correlation between the risk perception and age, with the over 75 perceiving a lower risk of getting infected compared to the younger participants. Our results should be taken as informative for future studies. Indeed, further studies on the older adults and the risk perception during emergencies are needed to better orient both communication and supporting strategies.

Introduction

The Coronavirus disease 2019 (COVID-19) deeply affected the daily living of people all over the world as many governments settled several rules and restrictions to limit the contagion. Indeed, at the end of 2019, after several cases of respiratory infections in the city of Wuhan of Hubei province in China, the city was locked down (J. Wu et al., 2020), and many countries adopted the same measure.

At the time of writing the present article, on the 30th of May 2020, there were 5.8 million infected cases all over the world, and Italy counted 232,664 confirmed cases becoming one of the first countries for the spread of the infection, with the Lombardy region as the most affected area within Italy (88,758 cases). As a consequence, the Italian government imposed a series of restrictions consisting of social distancing, the prohibition of all gathering activities, and confinement measures. Moreover, some guidelines concerning the behaviors to adopt were settled to prevent the infection spread, such as frequently washing the hands, wearing the mask, and avoiding public places. Compliance with these restrictions is of primary importance, especially for the protection of the most vulnerable categories of the population, including older adults.

Given the higher risk associated with the infection for this category of the population, it is important to consider that the current emergency could impact the perceived risk of getting infected which can bring, in turn, important consequences (Le Couteur et al., 2020; Yuan et al., 2020). As a matter of fact, previous studies highlighted the relationship between risk perception and psychological wellbeing, especially for people who are in quarantine and in high-risk areas (Chong et al., 2004; X. Liu et al., 2012; M. Liu et al., 2020; P. Wu et al., 2009); furthermore, despite heterogeneous results, it is well known the existence of a strict link between the risk perception and the adoption of health behaviors (Carlucci et al., 2020). For instance, a study carried out during the Severe Acute Respiratory Syndrome (SARS) outbreak highlighted the reduction of the perceived risk of getting infected while adopting precautionary actions (Brug et al., 2004). Conversely, a recent study conducted during the COVID-19 pandemic reported a decrease of protective behaviors in those who show a lower perceived risk of contracting the virus (Pasion et al., 2020). In any case, the perceived risk can affect the ways people adopt to react to the current emergency (Carlucci et al., 2020), so that exploring the risk perception within the population could be very informative for adjusting the policies adopted by the governments.

Risk perception has been widely explored in many different contexts, and the literature produced so far highlights the influence of both demographic and social factors on risk perception (Lanciano et al., 2020; Weber et al., 2002). Specifically, it seems to decrease as age increases (Bruine de Bruin, 2020; Pasion et al., 2020) and it has been described as higher in women than men (Gustafson, 1998; Harris & Jenkins, 2006). Lower risk perception has been reported in older than younger adults during both H5N1 and COVID-19 epidemics (Fielding et al., 2005; Pasion et al., 2020). Furthermore, the social proximity with people affected by the virus can affect the risk perception as well; for instance, a study found the persons who knew someone infected with COVID-19 perceiving higher risk and more anxious thoughts than the others (M. Liu et al., 2020). Notwithstanding this evidence, very few studies analyzed whether the risk perception' influencing factors hold when considering only the older segment of the population.

Moreover, given the global reach of the current COVID-19 pandemic along with the governments' need to timely communicate the adoption of preventive measures to all the population, it is worth considering the weight the sources of information have in determining the perceived risk associated with COVID-19. As well-pointed-out by Siebenhaar et al. (2020), if it is true that exposure to epidemic-related information can lead to appropriate risk perception (Garfin et al., 2020), it is also true that excessive and/or inconsistent information can cause negative feelings about the perceived risk for health conditions (Cava et al., 2005). A recent study by M. Liu et al. (2020) showed that media exposure to information about COVID-19 has played a crucial role in increasing the risk perception and anxiety of the public during the pandemic (M. Liu et al., 2020). Most of the studies focused mainly on the effects different information' contents have on risk perception (see, for instance, Olagoke et al., 2020) and less on the sources they derived from (see, for instance, Zhong et al., 2020), and none explored their relationship with the perceived risk of older adults, to our knowledge.

Given the paucity of studies focused on how older adults perceived the risk related to COVID-19, we aimed at exploring the risk perception of contracting COVID-19 and the related factors in the aging population in Italy, with a focus on the Lombardy region during the peak of the emergency. Due to the exploratory nature of the study, we think our results can give useful hints for orienting future studies targeting the most vulnerable categories of the population, such as older adults.

Methods

Sample

Between the 16th of March and the 17th of April 2020, we enrolled 514 participants older than 60 (mean age ± SD: 71.44 ± 5.41; 288 female) either formally belonging to older adults' associations or informally related to them. All the participants resided in the Lombardy region of Italy. We excluded participants who did not speak and correctly understand the Italian language, who were not cognitively competent, as well as participants who had language impairments, i.e., reading comprehension impairments. Informed consent was obtained prior to participation in the study through an online form. The study was designed according to the ethical standards of the Declaration of Helsinki and it received approval from the ethical committee of the Fondazione IRCCS Istituto Neurologico Carlo Besta of Milan.

Instruments

All the participants were administered with an online structured ad-hoc socio-demographic questionnaire to collect socio-demographic and personal information including the occupational status, health conditions, number of persons living with the participants, city where the participants are living, knowledge of persons affected by the COVID-19.

Furthermore, a series of ad-hoc items were administered to collect information about the (i) risk perception, (ii) sources of information used to be informed about COVID-19 emergency, and (iii) actions taken to avoid contracting the COVID-19.

Specifically, for the risk perception, we used some of the items described in the study by Brug et al. (2004) during the SARS epidemics in the Netherlands by asking participants to rate on a Likert scale from 1 (i.e., very little) to 5 (i.e., very much) the perceived risk of either contracting the COVID-19 or other potential threats (see Table 4 for a full list of the items).

As for the sources of information mostly used by participants, they had to indicate which source/s of information they used to stay updated on the COVID-19 emergency among the followings: Television, journals, magazines, internet, relatives, friends, medical doctors, and other health professionals (e.g., nurses, pharmacist).

Finally, to collect information about the actions taken to avoid getting infected, we selected 16 items out of 18 used in the study by Brug et al. (2004) by asking participants to indicate every action undertaken since the start of the emergency in Italy (Table 3). Differently from Brug et al. (2004), we did not consider the item "Use disinfectants" as we thought that this item was very similar to "Pay more attention to cleansing", furthermore, we did not consider the item "Do not go to school and work" as the Italian government had already restricted these activities also before the start of the interviews. All the participants answered by considering the period from the beginning of the outbreak in Italy (21st of February 2020); this reference period was chosen because, at the time of the interviews (from 16th of March to 17th of April), the Italian government already imposed the lockdown, and it represented the only way to explore which actions have been undertaken to avoid to getting infected.

Statistical analyses

Data have been analyzed by using Statistical Package for Social Science (IBM® SPSS® Statistic, Version 20). Descriptive statistics were reported either as mean ± standard deviation or as frequencies (see also Tables 1–3).

The perceived risk of contracting COVID-19 has been considered as a dependent variable of interest. Firstly, we performed a Friedman test to explore if there was a significant difference in perceiving the risk of contracting COVID-19 and the risk associated with other threats. Then, we ran separate Wilcoxon signed-rank tests on the different combinations of related variables to explore where the difference occurred.

Furthermore, we explored if there was a relationship between the perceived risk of contracting COVID-19 and the total number of both sources of information used and actions undertaken to avoid getting infected by performing two separate Spearman's correlations. We also explored the correlation between actions undertaken and the total number of sources of information as the Italian government has extensively used the media to communicate the preventive behaviors to adopt.

Finally, we explored if there was any difference in the perceived risk of contracting COVID-19 depending on factors significantly related to the risk perception according to what has been reported by the literature. Specifically, we explored whether a difference in the perceived risk of contracting COVID-19 was related to gender, age, and social factors, namely knowing persons who contracted the virus and living alone. For this purpose, we performed a series of Mann–Whitney tests to compare men with women, who reported to know infected persons with who reported to do not know infected persons, and who declared to live alone with who declared to live with someone else. For the factor age, we performed a Spearman's correlation between the perceived risk of contracting COVID-19 and the individuals' age in years.

Alpha level was set at $p < .05$ for all the analyses. Bonferroni correction for multiple comparisons has been applied whenever necessary.

Results

Most of the sample (91.8%) was composed of retired people; the years from the beginning of retirement were 11.94 on average (SD = 9.09). As high as 75.6% of the sample was living with someone at the time of the interview (number of individuals living with ranged from 1 to 5). Furthermore, most of the participants (55.8%) declared to suffer from chronic pathologies mainly consisting of cardiovascular diseases (59.9%). See Table 1 for a complete overview of the main features of the sample.

Globally, the participants used, on average, four different sources of information to be informed about the COVID-19 emergency; the greatest percentage of participants (95.3%) declared to get information through television whilst few participants declared to stay informed also by means of both magazines (11%) and health professionals (18.4%; see the Table 2).

Table 1. The table shows the main sociodemographic features of the sample. Both percentages and total number of participants for each variable are shown in second column.

Educational level	% (n)
Elementary school	5.6 (29)
High school	23.1 (119)
Secondary school	38.1 (196)
Graduation	29.3 (151)
Post-graduation	3.3 (17)
None	0.3 (2)
Province	
Bergamo	4.6 (24)
Brescia	3.5 (18)
Como	0.7 (4)
Cremona	5.0 (26)
Lecco	3.5 (18)
Lodi	1.1 (6)
Mantova	5.2 (27)
Milano	53.8 (277)
Monza-Brianza	4.6 (24)
Pavia	3.1 (16)
Sondrio	2.1 (11)
Varese	12.2 (63)
Occupational Status	
Retired	91.8 (472)
Employed	4.2 (22)
Home-worker	3.1 (16)
Unemployed	0.7 (4)
Health Condition	
Presence of pathologies	55.8 (287)
Absence of pathologies	44.1 (227)
Connection with who contracted COVID-19	
Yes	40.2 (207)
No	59.7 (307)

Table 2. Percentage and total number of participants using (second column) or not (third column) specific source of information.

Source of information	Yes % (n)	No % (n)
Television	95.3 (490)	4.6 (24)
Internet	76.4 (393)	23.5 (121)
Relatives	74.7 (384)	25.2 (130)
Friends	69.2 (356)	30.7 (158)
Journals	58.5 (301)	41.4 (213)
Doctors	35.6 (183)	64.3 (331)
Health professionals	18.4 (95)	81.5 (419)
Magazines	11.0 (57)	88.9 (457)

As for the actions undertaken to avoid getting infected, the participants carried out, on average, 13 actions out of the 16 included in the present study (Table 3).

Table 3. Percentage and total number of participants who undertaken (second column) or not (third column) specific action to avoid getting infected by COVID-19.

Action	Yes % (n)	No % (n)
Avoiding aggregations	97.4 (501)	2.5 (13)
Avoiding handshakes	97.2 (500)	2.7 (14)
Washing the hands frequently	97.0 (499)	2.9 (15)
Avoiding infectious areas	95.9 (493)	4.0 (21)
Avoiding traveling with aeroplane	95.3 (490)	4.6 (24)
Avoiding eating in restaurants	92.9 (478)	7.0 (36)
Avoiding eating in shopping centers	92.4 (475)	7.5 (39)
Avoiding traveling with taxi	91.2 (469)	8.7 (45)
Eating healthy food	90.6 (466)	9.3 (48)
Avoiding using public transport	90.4 (465)	9.5 (49)
Paying more attention to cleansing	85.9 (442)	14.0 (72)
Sufficiently sleeping	78.4 (403)	21.5 (111)
Wearing the mask	74.5 (383)	25.5 (131)
Avoiding specific kind of people	64.2 (330)	35.7 (184)
Practicing more physical exercise	63.2 (325)	36.7 (189)
Taking dietary supplements	24.9 (128)	75.0 (386)

Table 4. Wilcoxon signed-rank test results on risk perception. For every comparison (first column) both Z and *p* values are reported.

Comparison	Z	p-value
COVID19-Cancer[b**]	−11.45	<.001
COVID19-Common flu[b**]	−4.3	<.001
COVID19-Domestic accidents[a]	−.24	.807
COVID19-Road accidents[a]	−.25	.8
COVID19-Food poisoning[a**]	−3.46	<.001
Cancer-Common flu[b**]	−7.87	<.001
Cancer-Domestic accidents[b**]	−11.23	<.001
Cancer-Road accidents[a**]	−11.25	<.001
Cancer-Food poisoning[a**]	−12.93	<.001
Common flu-Domestic accidents[a**]	−4.27	<.001
Common flu-Road accidents[a**]	−4.39	<.001
Common flu-Food poisoning[a**]	−7.52	<.001
Domestic accidents-Road accidents[b]	−.32	.74
Domestic accidents-Food poisoning[a**]	−4.46	<.001
Road accidents-Food poisoning[a**]	−5.29	<.001

[a]Based on positive ranks; [b]Based on negative ranks; **Significant result after Bonferroni correction.

Perceived risk of contracting COVID-19 vs other threats

There was a statistically significant difference in the perceived risk depending on different threats ($\chi^2_{(5)}$ = 333.8; $p < .001$). Specifically, the perceived risk of contracting COVID-19 was lower than the perceived risk of having common flu (Z = −4.3; $p < .001$) and cancer (Z = −11.45; $p < .001$), and it was higher than the perceived risk associated with food poisoning (Z = −3.46; $p = .001$). The perceived risk associated with common flu was significantly higher than all the other threats (all p-values<.001), except for cancer. Indeed, the perceived risk associated with cancer was higher than the perceived risk associated with common flu (Z = −7.87; $p < 001$) as well as than all the other threats (all p-values<.001). Conversely, the perceived risk associated with food poisoning was significantly lower than the perceived risk associated with all the other threats (all p-values<.001). Table 4 shows the results derived from multiple comparisons.

Relationship between the perceived risk of contracting COVID-19 and both sources of information and actions undertaken

A significant positive correlation was found between the perceived risk associated with COVID-19 and the total number of sources of information used by each participant (Spearman's $rho_{(514)}$ = .117; $p < .001$), whilst the correlation between the perceived risk of contracting COVID-19 and the total number of actions undertaken by each participant did not reach the significance (Spearman's $rho_{(514)}$ = −.021; p = .627). However, the number of actions undertaken was positively correlated to the number of sources of information (Spearman's rho $_{(514)}$ = .198; $p < .001$).

Gender difference on the perceived risk of contracting COVID-19

We did not find any difference when comparing the perceived risk of contracting COVID-19 between men and women (Z = −.625; p = .532).

Difference on the perceived risk of contracting COVID-19 due to social factors

No difference was found between individuals living alone and individuals living with someone else (Z = −.673; p = .501). Conversely, the perceived risk of contracting COVID-19 was higher in who declared to know infected persons (mean rank = 275.28) compared to who declared to do not know infected persons (mean rank = 245.51; Z = −2.32; p = .02).

Age difference on the perceived risk of contracting COVID-19

We found a significant negative correlation between the age and the perceived risk of contracting COVID-19 (Spearman's $rho_{(514)}$ = .-113; p = .003). Thus, we further explored this pattern by dividing our sample by age-classes identifying three different groups, namely the youngest-old (from 60 to 69 years), middle-old (from 70 to 74 years), and the oldest-old (75+ years). We then performed a Kruskal–Wallis test attesting a significant difference between groups on the perceived risk of contracting COVID-19 ($\chi^2_{(2)}$ = 14.35; p = .001). The post-hoc test revealed a higher risk perception in the youngest-old (mean rank = 189.28) compared to the oldest-old (mean rank = 148.78; Z = −3.76; $p < .001$), and a similar trend when comparing the middle-old (mean rank = 156.89) to the oldest-old (mean rank = 134.07; Z = −2.37; p = .017).

Discussion

As attested by previous studies carried-out during epidemics, older adults are considered vulnerable and with a high risk for their health (K. Liu et al., 2020; Mehra et al., 2020; Wang et al., 2020). As the risk perception is strictly linked to both psychological wellbeing and adherence to quarantine protocols (Carlucci et al., 2020; M. Liu et al., 2020), it is relevant exploring risk perception and the related factors already documented in the literature (Brug et al., 2004; Zhang & Feei Ma, 2020) also in the older segment of the population. With this aim, we explored the risk perception of getting infected by COVID-19 in a sample of people older than 60 years residing in the Lombardy region of Italy during the emergency of the COVID-19 pandemic.

Despite the fact that COVID-19 has been described as much more dangerous than the common flu, especially for older adults, the perceived risk of contracting the virus was lower than the perceived risk associated with other threats such as common flu and cancer. Our result is in line with a previous study exploring the perceived risk associated with SARS in the Netherlands (Brug et al., 2004) and reporting higher risk perception related to common flu than SARS. These previous results are probably explicable with the low SARS diffusion in the Netherlands at the time of the study. To explain our results, instead, we have to take into account the strict link that does exist between risk perception and the perception of control (Brug et al., 2004); people feel themselves more at risk for threats they cannot control (Frewer et al., 1994; Källmén, 2000; Klein & Kunda, 1994; Nordgren et al., 2007). We think that, in our study, the lower perceived risk of getting COVID-19 is linked to lockdown, a situation in which people are confined at home where they feel safer and protected from contracting the virus. Furthermore, our sample was not worried about home accidents and falls, despite age-related mobility limitations, thus confirming that they did perceive their home as safe (Hughes et al., 2008; Martins et al., 2016). Overall, our results on risk perception related to COVID-19 are in line with other studies on older adults during the COVID-19 pandemic showing how this segment of the population perceived a lower risk of getting infected (Bruine de Bruin, 2020), and better reacted to the stressful situation (Pearman et al., 2020) than the rest of the population.

Although we did not compare older adults with younger individuals, we found the oldest individuals, i.e., the oldest-old group, perceiving a lower risk of contracting COVID-19 compared to the youngest ones, i.e., youngest- and middle-old groups. This result is in line with other studies conducted during the epidemics that reported a decrease in risk perception in the oldest-old (Fielding et al., 2005; Pasion et al., 2020). A possible explanation for this phenomenon could lie in the decrease of the fear of death with the age increase; in other words, the oldest-old group may be less worried about contracting an illness, and, therefore, shows a lower risk perception (Bruine de Bruin, 2020; Pasion et al., 2020). A complementary explanation concerns the decline in the executive functions in aging (Giorgio et al., 2010), as they underlie risk perception and risk-taking (Capone et al., 2016). What is worth highlighting, embracing both psychological and cognitive explanations, is the lower perceived risk in the older segment of the population which can bring important consequences, being the risk perception strictly related with the compliance to the quarantine protocols (Carlucci et al., 2020).

As previous studies attested that social factors could affect the risk perception and the behaviors adopted during the emergencies (see, for instance, M. Liu et al., 2020), it is of uttermost importance considering these factors when studying older adults. Indeed, this segment of the population is frequently disadvantaged due to the lack of strong social networking, a factor that can increase the sense of loneliness, fear, and risk perception (Parlapani et al., 2020; Yu et al., 2020). However, the only difference we found when taking into account social factors, namely living with someone and knowing persons who contracted the COVID-19, was related to higher risk perception in who have had direct experience of other persons contracting the virus. This result is in line with the study of Liu et al. (M. Liu et al., 2020) in which social proximity to COVID-19 was positively associated with anxiety. Probably, having direct experience of someone that contracted COVID-19 makes people perceive the risk of infection as closer and more real.

Finally, the sources of information play an important role during emergencies as they can greatly affect the risk perception and its related feelings (Cava et al., 2005; Garfin et al., 2020). Since previous studies strengthened the link between risk perception and emergency-related information (Garfin et al., 2020; Olagoke et al., 2020; Siebenhaar et al., 2020), we here explored if this factor influenced the older adults' risk perception as well. We found an increase in risk perception with the increase in the number of sources of information used. Different studies already outlined the impact of the infodemic on risk perception and mental well-being during the epidemics (Cava et al., 2005; Doraiswamy et al., 2020; Huang & Zhao, 2020): sometimes media information can be unclear and discordant, and this could lead to uncertainty and uneven compliance with quarantine protocols. Here, we want to strengthen the importance of focusing not only on the contents of the information but also on the amount of information, as our result referred to the number of sources of information used. In line with this finding, another research study conducted during the COVID-19 pandemic (M. Liu et al., 2020) reported an increase in anxiety due to the continuous exposure to pandemic-related information, also considering that in the context of an emergency many people, in addition to actively seeking news, receive information also in a passive manner. Taken together, this evidence suggests to tailor communication strategies to the older adults' needs during emergencies.

In Italy, the mainstream media following WHO and Government authorities' indications have played also an important role in indicating good practices to adopt to avoid the contagion, such as avoiding aggregations, washing hands, wearing mask. This could have helped our sample to follow the guidelines, even before some of these behaviors had become mandatory. Indeed, in our study, participants put into action most of the possible behaviors aimed to avoid contracting the COVID-19, and, contrary to what could be expected, these behaviors did not correlate with the perceived risk of getting infected. Since the beginning of the pandemic, the Italian government relied on the main media to timely communicate the preventive measures to adopt, so it is plausible to hypothesize a relation between the preventive behaviors and the information spread; as a matter of fact, we found a positive correlation between these factors. Future studies should better analyze the relations between risk perception, information, and preventive behaviors by adopting different statistical models, such as moderator and mediator analyses.

All the present results could be considered preliminary and not generalizable to the general population as our sample is biased by the recruitment procedure. Indeed, we recruited people belonging or close to older adults' associations who are probably well-integrated in the society, with strong social relations, thus being less at risk of isolation and more sustained in facing the situation compared to the general older adults' population. Secondly, since we focused on a new, unexpected, and emerging theme, we are aware that in the progression of the pandemic there will be an increase of publications; thus, the picture could not be complete yet.

To our knowledge, no research gave relevance to how older adults perceived, lived, and reacted to the COVID-19 emergency in Italy yet. This exploratory study investigated the risk perception of Italian older adults during the peak of the COVID-19 emergency. Based on these preliminary results, future studies could deeply explore the factors related to risk perception also considering the different phases of the emergency. Indeed, the present study focused mainly on the lockdown phase at the beginning of the emergency, highlighting the need to take into account the risk perception of older adults as it affects the way people adopt to cope with the situation and their well-being. Studying risk perception in aging population becomes fundamental during emergencies to better orient the communication strategies as well as the social and health policies that should mainly ground on the needs of this category of the population.

Acknowledgments

Authors would like to thank all the participants that took part in the study.

ORCID

Claudia Toppo ⓘ http://orcid.org/0000-0002-1312-6679

Declaration of interest

The authors have no conflicts of interest.

References

Brug, J., Aro, A. R., Oenema, A., De Zwart, O., Richardus, J. H., & Bishop, G. D. (2004). SARS risk perception, knowledge, precautions, and information sources, the Netherlands. *Emerging Infectious Diseases, 10*(8), 1486–1489. https://doi.org/10.3201/eid1008.040283

Bruine de Bruin, W. (2020). Age differences in COVID-19 risk perceptions and mental health: Evidence from a national US survey conducted in March 2020. *The Journals of Gerontology. Series B, Psychological Sciences and Social Sciences.* Advance online publication. https://doi.org/10.1093/geronb/gbaa074

Capone, F., Capone, G., Di Pino, G., Florio, L., Oricchio, G., & Di Lazzaro, V. (2016). Linking cognitive abilities with the propensity for risk-taking: The balloon analogue risk task. *Neurological Sciences, 37*(12), 2003–2007. https://doi.org/10.1007/s10072-016-2721-8

Carlucci, L., D'ambrosio, I., & Balsamo, M. (2020). Demographic and attitudinal factors of adherence to quarantine guidelines during covid-19: The italian model. *Frontiers in Psychology, 11*(October), 1–13. https://doi.org/10.3389/fpsyg.2020.559288

Cava, M. A., Fay, K. E., Beanlands, H. J., McCay, E. A., & Wignall, R. (2005). Risk perception and compliance with quarantine during the SARS outbreak. *Journal of Nursing Scholarship, 37*(4), 343–347. https://doi.org/10.1111/j.1547-5069.2005.00059.x

Chong, M. Y., Wang, W. C., Hsieh, W. C., Lee, C. Y., Chiu, N. M., Yeh, W. C., Huang, T. L., Wen, J. K., & Chen, C. L. (2004). Psychological impact of severe acute respiratory syndrome on health workers in a tertiary hospital. *British Journal of Psychiatry, 185*(AUG.), 127–133. https://doi.org/10.1192/bjp.185.2.127

Doraiswamy, S., Cheema, S., & Mamtani, R. (2020). Older people and epidemics: A call for empathy. *Age and Ageing, 49*(3), 493–493. https://doi.org/10.1093/ageing/afaa060

Fielding, R., Lam, W. W. T., Ho, E. Y. Y., Lam, T. H., Hedley, A. J., & Leung, G. M. (2005). Avian influenza risk perception, Hong Kong. *Emerging Infectious Diseases, 11*(5), 677–682. https://doi.org/10.3201/eid1105.041225

Frewer, L. J., Shepherd, R., & Sparks, P. (1994). The interrelationship between perceived knowledge, control and risk associated with a range of food-related hazards targeted at the individual, other people and society. *Journal of Food Safety, 14*(1), 19–40. https://doi.org/10.1111/j.1745-4565.1994.tb00581.x

Garfin, D. R., Silver, R. C., & Holman, E. A. (2020). The novel coronavirus (COVID-2019) outbreak: Amplification of public health consequences by media exposure. *Health Psychology, 39*(5), 355–357. https://doi.org/10.1037/hea0000875

Giorgio, A., Santelli, L., Tomassini, V., Bosnell, R., Smith, S., De Stefano, N., & Johansen-Berg, H. (2010). Age-related changes in grey and white matter structure throughout adulthood. *NeuroImage, 51*(3), 943–951. https://doi.org/10.1016/j.neuroimage.2010.03.004

Gustafson, P. E. (1998). Gender differences in risk perception: Theoretical and methodological perspectives. *Risk Analysis, 18*(6), 805–811. https://doi.org/10.1023/B:RIAN.0000005926.03250.c0

Harris, C. R., & Jenkins, M. (2006). Gender differences in risk assessment: Why do women take fewer risks than men? *Judgment and Decision Making*, *1*(1), 48–63. http://www.albacharia.ma/xmlui/bitstream/handle/123456789/31957/jdm06016.pdf?sequence=1

Huang, Y., & Zhao, N. (2020). Mental health burden for the public affected by the COVID-19 outbreak in China: Who will be the high-risk group? *Psychology, Health & Medicine*, 1–12. Advance online publication. https://doi.org/10.1080/13548506.2020.1754438

Hughes, K., van Beurden, E., Eakin, E. G., Barnett, L. M., Patterson, E., Backhouse, J., Jones, S., Hauser, D., Beard, J. R., & Newman, B. (2008). Older persons' perception of risk of falling: Implications for fall-prevention campaigns. *American Journal of Public Health*, *98*(2), 351–357. https://doi.org/10.2105/AJPH.2007.115055

Källmén, H. (2000). Manifest anxiety, general self-efficacy and locus of control as determinants of personal and general risk perception. *Journal of Risk Research*, *3*(2), 111–120. https://doi.org/10.1080/136698700376626

Klein, W. M., & Kunda, Z. (1994). Exaggerated self-assessments and the preference for controllable risks. *Organizational Behavior and Human Decision Processes*, *59*(3), 410–427. https://doi.org/10.1006/obhd.1994.1067

Lanciano, T., Graziano, G., Curci, A., Costadura, S., & Monaco, A. (2020). Risk perceptions and psychological effects during the Italian COVID-19 emergency. *Frontiers in Psychology*, *11*, 2434. https://doi.org/10.3389/fpsyg.2020.580053

Le Couteur, D. G., Anderson, R. M., & Newman, A. B. (2020). COVID-19 through the lens of gerontology. *The Journals of Gerontology: Series A*, *75*(9), 1804. https://doi.org/10.1093/gerona/glaa077

Liu, K., Chen, Y., Lin, R., & Han, K. (2020). Clinical features of COVID-19 in elderly patients: A comparison with young and middle-aged patients. *Journal of Infection*, *80*(6), e14–e18. https://doi.org/10.1016/j.jinf.2020.03.005

Liu, M., Zhang, H., & Huang, H. (2020). Media exposure to COVID-19 information, risk perception, social and geographical proximity, and self-rated anxiety in China. *BMC Public Health*, *20*(1), 1. https://doi.org/10.1186/s12889-020-09761-8

Liu, X., Kakade, M., Fuller, C. J., Fan, B., Fang, Y., Kong, J., Guan, Z., & Wu, P. (2012). Depression after exposure to stressful events: Lessons learned from the severe acute respiratory syndrome epidemic. *Comprehensive Psychiatry*, *53*(1), 15–23. https://doi.org/10.1016/j.comppsych.2011.02.003

Martins, L., Barkokébas, B., Baptista, J., & Arezes, P. (2016). Domestic safety and accidents risk perception by active elderly. *Advances in Intelligent Systems and Computing*, *491*, 285–295. https://doi.org/10.1007/978-3-319-41929-9_27

Mehra, A., Rani, S., Sahoo, S., Parveen, S., Singh, A. P., Chakrabarti, S., & Grover, S. (2020). A crisis for elderly with mental disorders: Relapse of symptoms due to heightened anxiety due to COVID-19. *Asian Journal of Psychiatry*, *51*(April), 102114. https://doi.org/10.1016/j.ajp.2020.102114

Nordgren, L. F., van der Pligt, J., & van Harreveld, F. (2007). Unpacking perceived control in risk perception: The mediating role of anticipated regret. *Journal of Behavioral Decision Making*, *20*(5), 533–544. https://doi.org/10.1002/bdm.565

Olagoke, A. A., Olagoke, O. O., & Hughes, A. M. (2020). Exposure to coronavirus news on mainstream media: The role of risk perceptions and depression. *British Journal of Health Psychology*, *25*(4), 865–874. https://doi.org/10.1111/bjhp.12427

Parlapani, E., Holeva, V., Nikopoulou, V. A., Sereslis, K., Athanasiadou, M., Godosidis, A., Stephanou, T., & Diakogiannis, I. (2020). Intolerance of uncertainty and loneliness in older adults during the COVID-19 pandemic. *Frontiers in Psychiatry*, *11*(August), 1–12. https://doi.org/10.3389/fpsyt.2020.00842

Pasion, R., Paiva, T. O., Fernandes, C., & Barbosa, F. (2020). The AGE effect on protective behaviors during the COVID-19 outbreak: Sociodemographic, perceptions and psychological accounts. *Frontiers in Psychology, 11*(October), 1–14. https://doi.org/10.3389/fpsyg.2020.561785

Pearman, A., Hughes, M. L., Smith, E. L., & Neupert, S. D. (2020). Age differences in risk and resilience factors in COVID-19-related stress. *The Journals of Gerontology Series B: Psychological Sciences and Social Sciences.* Advance online publication. https://doi.org/10.1093/geronb/gbaa120/5879986

Siebenhaar, K. U., Köther, A. K., & Alpers, G. W. (2020). Dealing with the COVID-19 infodemic: Distress by information, information avoidance, and compliance with preventive measures. *Frontiers in Psychology, 11*(November), 1–11. https://doi.org/10.3389/fpsyg.2020.567905

Wang, L., He, W., Yu, X., Hu, D., Bao, M., Liu, H., Zhou, J., & Jiang, H. (2020). Coronavirus disease 2019 in elderly patients: Characteristics and prognostic factors based on 4-week follow-up. *Journal of Infection, 80*(6), 639–645. https://doi.org/10.1016/j.jinf.2020.03.019

Weber, E. U., Blais, A. R., & Betz, N. E. (2002). A domain-specific risk-attitude scale: Measuring risk perceptions and risk behaviors. *Journal of Behavioral Decision Making, 15*(4), 263–290. https://doi.org/10.1002/bdm.414

Wu, J., Gamber, M., & Sun, W. (2020). Does Wuhan need to be in lockdown during the Chinese Lunar new year? *International Journal of Environmental Research and Public Health, 17*(3), 1002. https://doi.org/10.3390/ijerph17031002

Wu, P., Fang, Y., Guan, Z., Fan, B., Kong, J., Yao, Z., Liu, X., Fuller, C. J., Susser, E., Lu, J., & Hoven, C. W. (2009). The psychological impact of the SARS epidemic on hospital employees in China: Exposure, risk perception, and altruistic acceptance of risk. *Canadian Journal of Psychiatry, 54*(5), 302–311. https://doi.org/10.1177/070674370905400504

Yu, J., Choe, K., & Kang, Y. (2020). Anxiety of older persons living alone in the community. *Healthcare, 8*(3), 287. https://doi.org/10.3390/healthcare8030287

Yuan, Y., Wang, N., & Ou, X. (2020). Caution should be exercised for the detection of SARS-CoV-2, especially in the elderly. *Journal of Medical Virology, 92*(9), 1641–1648. https://doi.org/10.1002/jmv.25796

Zhang, Y., & Feei Ma, Z. (2020). Impact of the COVID-19 pandemic on mental health and quality of life among local residents in Liaoning Province, China: A cross-sectional study. *Mdpi.Com.* https://doi.org/10.3390/ijerph17072381

Zhong, Y., Liu, W., & Lee, T. (2020, January). *Since January 2020 Elsevier has created a COVID-19 resource centre with free information in English and Mandarin on the novel coronavirus COVID- 19. The COVID-19 resource centre is hosted on Elsevier Connect, the company ' s public news and information.*

Associations between Volunteering and Mental Health during COVID-19 among Chinese Older Adults

Wai Chan ⓘD, Cheryl Hiu Kwan Chui ⓘD, Johnson Chun Sing Cheung ⓘD, Terry Yat Sang Lum ⓘD and Shiyu Lu ⓘD

ABSTRACT

Evidence about the association between volunteering and the mental health of older adults during COVID-19 remains under-explored. This study investigated (1) patterns of volunteering among older adults in Hong Kong during COVID-19; (2) associations between volunteering and mental health of older adults during COVID-19; and (3) associations between key psychological resources (e.g., self-efficacy and self-esteem) and volunteering among older adults during COVID-19. This study applied a cross-sectional design with data collected from 128 older adults in June 2020, who were trained as volunteers in a volunteer program that began before COVID-19. The study found that older adults continued to actively contribute to their communities by engaging in volunteering during COVID-19. The specific type of volunteering activities was linked to few depressive and anxiety symptoms. Older adults with increased self-esteem prior to COVID-19 were more likely to participate in volunteering activities related to COVID-19. Our study suggested that encouraging older adults to volunteer during the pandemic is a key pathway to maintain mental health. Social workers are encouraged to engage older adults in volunteerism regularly to offset the risk of depression and anxiety symptoms in times of crisis.

Introduction

Physical distancing measures introduced to help control the spread of COVID-19 were one of many factors that contributed to mental health challenges during the pandemic (Holmes et al., 2020; Smith et al., 2020), particularly among older adults. People aged 50 and older who have chronic conditions have been advised to stay home and avoid gathering since they have a disproportionately higher infection and mortality rates of COVID-19 (Bonanad et al., 2020). It inevitably increases social isolation. Santini et al. (2020) found that social disconnectedness predicted higher depression and anxiety symptoms among older adults. As growing numbers of people are experiencing unprecedented adversity, it is imperative to place mental health at the center of global responses to and recovery from the pandemic (United Nations, 2020).

Promoting volunteering is one of the promising interventions to protect older adults' mental health amid COVID-19 (Holmes et al., 2020). Volunteering refers to unpaid non-compulsory activities undertaken by an individual either through an organization or directly for others' benefits (Morrow-Howell, 2010; Taniguchi, 2012). Volunteering has been found to be positively linked to physical and psychological well-being in older adults (Burr et al., 2015; Lum & Lightfoot, 2005; Russell et al., 2019). For example, Choi and Kim (2011) found that both volunteering and making any charitable donation have a positive effect on psychological well-being among older adults. Previous studies have identified potential underlying mechanisms linking volunteering and mental health for older adults, such as compensating for the loss of role following retirement, providing meaning to life, and maintaining social contact (Filges et al., 2020; Morrow-Howell, 2010). In particular, existing literature has found that volunteering is associated with the sense of control in later life (Drewelies et al., 2017), which is defined as the belief in having control of one's own life experience (Schulz & Heckhausen, 1999). People with a higher sense of control are less prone to depression in the face of adversity (Ryon & Gleason, 2014). The COVID-19 pandemic and containment strategies have produced widely shared feelings of anxiety and loss of control due to the abrupt disruption of people's daily routines and regular activities. Under such adverse constraints, volunteering could help older adults maintain good mental health.

However, little research has investigated whether older adults volunteer, and associations between volunteering and mental health during COVID-19. Although a recent study found an increase in informal volunteering in some countries during lockdown (Mak & Fancourt, 2020), it is unclear whether older adults who are at greater risk of infection and mortality in this pandemic volunteer. Only one recent study in Canada and the United States using a convenient sampling found that middle-aged and older adults engaged in more informal volunteering (e.g., emotional support) than other age groups during the pandemic (Sin et al., 2020). Their engagement in volunteering activities was associated with lower negative affects (e.g., angry and frustration) (Sin et al., 2020). However, there is limited evidence about how volunteering is associated with specific mental health problems such as depression and anxiety symptoms among older adults. Investigating the associations between volunteering and mental health among older adults during the COVID-19 pandemic can enrich our understanding of how older adults act for others and whether the psychological effects of volunteering can be maintained in times of crisis.

Findings generated from this study can provide evidence for developing strategies to reduce depression and anxiety among older adults during the pandemic.

Given the positive effects associated with volunteering among older adults, understanding its antecedents is imperative. Previous studies have identified factors associated with volunteering among older people based on different perspectives, such as institutional perspective (e.g., role flexibility in a volunteer capacity, training, and incentive provided by the organization) (Morrow-Howell et al., 2001; Tang et al., 2009). In addition, previous studies found that understanding factors associated with volunteering from resource perspective is essential: individuals' resources were found to be determinants of volunteering, such as financial resources (e.g., income, housing, cars etc.), human resources (e.g., physical and mental health, education, skills, training, experience), and social resources (e.g., social support and social networks) (Niebuur et al., 2018; Wu et al., 2018). In addition, self-efficacy and self-esteem could be the key psychological resources for individuals to volunteer (Afolabi, 2014; Afolabi & Alade, 2015). However, there is little understanding about whether self-efficacy and self-esteem are associated with older adults' volunteering during the pandemic. Self-efficacy refers to individuals' confidence in their ability to engage in the behavior required to produce the desired outcomes (Bandura, 1977). Self-esteem is defined as an overall evaluation of one's self-worth and having the strength of character to act responsibly toward others (Rosenberg, 1965). There is evidence indicating that enhancing older adults' self-efficacy through volunteer interventions leads to more volunteering (Jiang et al., 2020), but not much evidence elucidating the association between self-esteem and volunteering. Self-esteem may be an important yet overlooked antecedent. For instance, it was found that adolescents with higher self-esteem predicted more volunteer behavior (Afolabi, 2014). However, this association has not been explored among older adults. Understanding how self-efficacy and self-esteem are associated with volunteering in times of crisis can inform future intervention designs aimed at promoting volunteering among older adults.

In response, this study investigated: (1) the patterns of volunteering among older adults in Hong Kong during COVID-19; (2) the association between volunteering and mental health of older adults during COVID-19; and (3) the association between self-efficacy and self-esteem in determining volunteering among older adults during the pandemic. We hypothesized that (H1) older adults who volunteer have fewer depressive and anxiety symptoms during COVID-19, and (H2) older adults who have higher self-efficacy and self-esteem are more likely to volunteer during COVID-19.

Method

Sample

This study applied a cross-sectional design. Data were derived from the one-year follow-up assessment collected in June 2020 of 128 community-dwelling Chinese older adults in Hong Kong who participated in a single volunteer program. The program commenced before COVID-19 and was interrupted half-way by the outbreak in January 2020. To be eligible, participants needed to be aged 50 or older, fluent in Cantonese, and understand written Chinese. Participants were recruited from the elderly community centers. They were provided with health-related knowledge and skill training and were subsequently stationed at the centers in a voluntary capacity. However, no formal volunteer work was available from January 2020 onward as the centers were temporarily closed. A self-reported baseline assessment (T0) was conducted in June 2019, which included self-efficacy, self-esteem, and basic sociodemographic information. The self-reported follow-up assessment (T1) conducted in June 2020 additionally collected information about depression, anxiety, and participation in volunteering activities specifically related to COVID-19 since the outbreak of the pandemic (between January and June 2020). The study was reviewed and approved by the Human Research Ethics Committee, The University of Hong Kong.

Measures

Mental health

Depression symptoms were measured by the validated Chinese version of the Patient Health Questionnaire (PHQ-9) (Yeung et al., 2008). Scores range from 0 to 27, with higher scores indicating more depression symptoms. Cronbach's α was 0.89. Anxiety symptoms were measured by the validated Chinese version of the Generalized Anxiety Disorder 7-item scale (GAD-7) (Tong et al., 2016). Scores range from 0 to 21, with higher scores indicating more anxiety symptoms. Cronbach's α was 0.85.

Volunteering related to COVID-19

Participants were asked whether they had been engaged in the following volunteering activities related to COVID-19 since the outbreak of the pandemic, including (1) helping neighbors or friends to buy daily necessities, (2) helping neighbors or friends to buy facemasks, (3) helping neighbors or friends to buy pandemic prevention materials, (4) giving out facemasks, (5) giving out pandemic prevention materials, (6) taking care of neighbors' or friends' children, and (7) providing emotional support to neighbors or friends. We also asked participants whether they donated to a charity during the pandemic. Each item yielded an answer of "yes" (1) or "no" (0). Multiple response options were allowed. This measurement of participation in volunteering activities related to COVID-19 was created by the research team with extensive experience in productive aging research. The face validity was confirmed by clinical social workers and clinical psychologists.

Self-efficacy & self-esteem

Self-efficacy was measured by the Chinese version of the 10-item General Self-efficacy Scale (Zhang & Schwarzer, 1995). Scores range from 4 to 40, with higher scores indicating higher self-efficacy. Cronbach's α was 0.88. Self-esteem was measured by the Chinese version of Rosenberg's 10-item Global Self-esteem Scale (Cheng & Hamid, 1995). Scores range from 4 to 40, with higher scores indicating higher self-esteem. Cronbach's α was 0.79.

Sociodemographic variables

Participants were asked a series of questions related to their sociodemographic characteristics, including gender (male/female), age group (age 50–64/65 or above), the education level (primary and below/secondary/post-secondary), and marital status (married/others).

Analytic strategy

Descriptive statistics were used to summarize sample characteristics. To test whether volunteering among older adults is associated with fewer depressive and anxiety symptoms during COVID-19, we applied multivariate analysis using the generalized linear model (GLM). As a substantial number of participants scored zero on the PHQ-9 (48.4%) and GAD-7 (55.5%) and their distributions were skewed, the two dependent variables were transformed by adding one score to the raw data, respectively. GLM with a log-link function and gamma distribution was then applied for analysis, as suggested by previous studies (Fletcher et al., 2005; Manning et al., 2005).

To test whether older adults who have higher self-efficacy and self-esteem are more likely to volunteer during COVID-19, logistic regression analyses were conducted to examine the associations between self-efficacy and self-esteem at T1. Noting that the formal volunteer program starting before COVID-19 may increase self-efficacy and self-esteem, changes between T0 and T1 were also taken into account in this analysis. Changes in self-efficacy were recoded into three groups: participants with decreased self-efficacy (0), participants with no change in self-efficacy (1), and participants with increased self-efficacy (2). Likewise, changes in self-esteem were also recoded into three groups: decreased self-esteem (0), no change (1), and increased self-esteem (2). Additional analyses were conducted to identify any significant increases in self-efficacy and self-esteem between T0 and T1.

All sociodemographic variables were controlled for in the multivariate analysis using GLM and logistic regression. Statistical analyses were performed using SPSS 26.0 and Stata 15.1. Estimates with a *p*-value smaller than .05 were interpreted as statistically significant.

Results

Participants' characteristics and volunteering activities during the pandemic are presented in Table 1. The mean age of participants was 64.9 (SD = 6.80), about one-third of whom were aged 65 or older. Most were female (79.7%). Over half had completed secondary education (52.3%) and were married (60.9%). During the pandemic, they had a mean PHQ-9 score of 1.68 (SD = 2.73) and a mean GAD-7 score of 1.38 (SD = 2.26), indicating a low severity of depression and anxiety symptoms. Most engaged in at least one of volunteering activities (77.3%), such as providing emotional support to neighbors/ friends (69.5%) and giving facemasks to people in need (44.5%). Around one-third assisted neighbors/friends to purchase facemasks (32.0%) and pandemic prevention materials (26.6%) and giving pandemic prevention materials to people in need (29.7%). A few assisted neighbors/friends to purchase daily

Table 1. Sociodemographic characteristics (N = 128).

	%/Mean (Standard Deviation, SD)
Female	79.7
Age	64.9 (6.80)
50–64	68.8
65 or above	31.3
Education Level	
Primary and below	7.8
Secondary	52.3
Post-secondary	39.8
Marital Status	
Married	60.9
Others (Single/widowed/divorced/separated)	39.1
PHQ-9	1.68 (2.73)
GAD-7	1.38 (2.26)
Volunteering related to COVID-19	
Volunteering activities (any type listed below)	77.3
Assisting neighbors/friends to purchase daily necessities (e.g., canned food, rice, tissues) [a]	17.2
Assisting neighbors/friends to purchase facemasks [a]	32.0
Assisting neighbors/friends to purchase pandemic prevention materials (e.g., alcohol sanitizer, bleach) [a]	26.6
Taking care of neighbors'/friends' children [a]	3.9
Giving facemasks to people in need [a]	44.5
Giving pandemic prevention materials to people in need [a]	29.7
Providing emotional support to neighbors/friends [a]	69.5
Others [a]	11.7
Donating money	18.8

Notes: [a] Multiple responses allowed; PHQ-9 = Patient Health Questionnaire-9; GDA-7 = Generalized Anxiety Disorder-7; Other volunteering activities included sewing cloth facemasks and delivering meals to people in need.

Table 2. GLM for PHQ-9 and GAD-7 (N = 128).

	PHQ-9		GAD-7	
	Coefficient	SE	Coefficient	SE
Aged 65 or above (ref.: Below 65)	−0.15	0.19	0.01	0.19
Male (ref.: Female)	−0.09	0.19	−0.30	0.20
Married (ref.: Single/widowed/divorced/separated)	0.26	0.18	0.10	0.17
Education level (ref.: Primary and below)				
Secondary	0.15	0.26	0.30	0.29
Post-secondary	0.09	0.27	0.22	0.30
Volunteering activities				
Assisting others to purchase daily necessities	−0.41*	0.20	−0.36*	0.16
Constant	0.88**	0.26	0.68*	0.31
AIC	4.02		3.79	

Notes: AIC = The Akaike information criterion; PHQ-9 = Patient Health Questionnaire-9; GDA-7 = Generalized Anxiety Disorder-7. The GLM analyses for PHQ-9 and GAD-7 with other volunteering activities during COVID-19 can be provided upon request. SE = Standard Error.
*p < .05. **p < .01.

necessities (17.2%) and took care of children (3.9%). Some donated money (18.8%).

Table 2 shows the GLM results for the associations between volunteering activities and PHQ-9 and GAD-7. After controlling for age group, gender, marital status, and educational level, only helping others purchase daily necessities was negatively and significantly associated with PHQ-9 (β = −0.41, p = .039) and GAD-7 (β = −0.36, p = .027). It indicates that those engaged in this specific volunteering activity had fewer depressive symptoms and lower anxiety levels. We also tested the associations between other listed

Table 3. Logistic regression for specific volunteering activity (assisting others to purchase daily necessities) during COVID-19 (N = 128).

	Model 1			Model 2		
	OR	95% CI	p-value	OR	95% CI	p-value
Aged 65 or above (ref.: Below 65)	1.34	0.43–4.21	.612	0.93	0.28–3.04	.899
Male (ref.: Female)	0.80	0.20–3.11	.724	0.74	0.18–3.08	.674
Married (ref.: Single/widowed/divorced/separated)	1.01	0.37–3.15	.892	1.81	0.58–5.64	.310
Education level (ref.: Primary and below)						
Secondary	0.21	0.04–1.04	.055	0.25	0.06–1.13	.072
Post-secondary	0.19	0.04–1.00	.049	0.21	0.04–1.11	.067
Self-efficacy at T1	0.89	0.74–1.06	.189			
Changes in self-efficacy (T1-T0) (ref.: decreased self-efficacy)						
No change	0.25	0.03–2.31	.222			
Increased self-efficacy	2.23	0.69–7.19	.179			
Self-esteem at T1				1.03	0.87–1.22	.725
Changes in self-esteem (T1-T0) (ref.: decreased self-esteem)						
No change				3.89	0.63–24.21	.145
Increased self-esteem				8.09	1.47–44.61	.016
Constant	21.33		.296	0.72		.352
Likelihood ratio chi-square (8)	13.87		.085	16.85		.032
Pseudo R-square	0.17			0.21		

Notes: OR = odd ratio; CI = confidence interval. The logistic regression for other volunteering activities during COVID-19 can be provided upon request.

volunteering activities during COVID-19 with PHQ-9 and GAD-7, respectively. No significant association was found.

Table 3 shows the associations between the level of self-efficacy/self-esteem during COVID-19, changes in self-efficacy/self-esteem, and the specific volunteering activities: assisting neighbors/friends to purchase daily necessities during COVID-19. Only the logistic regression model for self-esteem fits the data ($\chi 2$ (8) = 16.85, p < .05, pseudo R-squared = 0.21). Controlling for covariates, we only found that participants with increased self-esteem between T0 and T1 were more likely to assist others to purchase daily necessities during COVID-19 (OR = 8.09, p = .016). We did not find any association between the level of self-efficacy and self-esteem measured during COVID-19 or changes in self-efficacy with volunteering activities related to assisting neighbors/friends to purchase daily necessities. Moreover, no associations were found between the levels of self-efficacy/self-esteem during the pandemic (T1) and changes in the levels of self-efficacy/self-esteem with other volunteering activities. Additional analysis found that self-efficacy and self-esteem significantly increased between T0 and T1 (Supplementary Table 1).

Discussion

This study aimed to understand older adults' participation in volunteering activities, investigate the associations between volunteering and depressive and anxiety symptoms among older adults, and examine whether older adults who have higher self-efficacy and self-esteem are more likely to volunteer during COVID-19. Three key findings were generated from this study: (1) older adults actively contributed to their communities by engaging in different volunteering activities during COVID-19; (2) that specific volunteering activity was linked to fewer depressive and anxiety symptoms among older adults; and (3) older adults with enhanced self-esteem before COVID-19 were more likely to volunteer during the pandemic. Additional insights can be generated from our study.

First, we found that most middle-aged and older adults remained active in providing different means of support to others during the pandemic. The majority of our sample engaged in at least one volunteering activity (77.3%). Among them, 69.5% provided emotional support to neighbors/friends, nearly half gave out facemasks to people in need, and 17.2% assisted others to purchase daily necessities.

Older adults' active engagement in volunteering activities, such as providing emotional support and giving out facemasks to people in need, reflects how civil society was mobilized and responded to the pandemic in Hong Kong. A series of bottom-up and self-initiated volunteering activities have been observed in Hong Kong's civil society (Wan et al., 2020). For instance, facemask sharing actions were initiated by local NGOs, shop owners, and individuals. People used social media platforms, such as Facebook and YouTube, to exchange COVID-related news, verify the facts, and show how to test unsatisfactory facemasks. NGOs and individuals held online workshops to teach how to make cloth facemasks and hand sanitizers at home. Such self-initiated, self-help and mutual help responses in civil society not only prevented a large-scale community outbreak in the early stages of the COVID-19 (Wan et al., 2020) but also presented many opportunities for capable older adults, motivating them to help others and contribute to their communities. In this regard, the influence of older adults who are capable and willing to contribute should not be overlooked.

Second, the study found that older adults who volunteered had fewer depressive and anxiety symptoms during COVID-19. This finding is aligned with existing literature that shows positive associations between helping others and mental health outcomes among older adults (Burr et al., 2015; Lum & Lightfoot, 2005; Russell et al., 2019). This finding further extends the existing literature by lending support that such benefits can still be maintained during a public health crisis.

However, we found that only one specific volunteering activity – assisting others to purchase daily necessities – was associated with better mental health outcomes, whereas no other association was found between other volunteering activities and mental health. Such findings may be explained by the nature of the volunteering activities if it is challenging and meaningful. The supply of facemasks and other pandemic prevention materials was tight and sold at sky-high prices in Hong Kong in the early stages of the pandemic. Facemasks became inaccessible for low-income families and expensive for most citizens, including older adults in our program. Giving out the facemasks to people in need could be meaningful but in fact, presents a high cost to older adults. Providing emotional support is important, yet it could be one of the regular components in voluntary activities in normal times. In contrast, assisting others to purchase daily necessities may be challenging but achievable for older adults since this kind of support is non-routine, requires skills of problem identification and demonstrates knowledge of their local neighborhoods but remaining within their ability. It has been suggested that older adults involved in challenging yet meaningful volunteering may benefit more (Chambré, 1993). Thus, it is plausible that older adults who volunteered exhibit fewer depressive and anxiety symptoms because such meaningful volunteer engagement provides greater contentment for older adults.

However, as previous studies suggested that older adults with more resources (e.g., wealth, health, skills, social support, and social network) are more likely to volunteer, it is also possible that those older adult volunteers may have more resources to cope with the stress and maintain their mental health during the pandemic than those without comparable resources. Therefore, the civil society and elderly services providers need to pay attention to equity and inclusion implication in organizing these activities, by matching the volunteering activities with older adults' resources and capacities, offering adequate education and training for older adult volunteers with low levels of resources, mingling older adult with different levels of resources in participating volunteering activities to strengthen their social ties and networks.

Third, we did not find any significant association between self-efficacy and self-esteem and volunteering in our study. It contrasts with our hypotheses and these previous studies, which have shown that volunteer participation was higher for people with higher self-esteem (Allen & Rushton, 1983), while low self-esteem has been linked to lower levels of volunteerism among young people (Afolabi, 2014). We only found that self-efficacy and self-esteem were enhanced during COVID-19, even though the program was disrupted by COVID-19. Our volunteer program possibly increased older adults' overall evaluation of self-worth and confidence in helping others even in difficult times. It is also possible that participation in our volunteer program and helping others during adverse times jointly increased the self-esteem and self-efficacy of older adults. The causal relationship between self-esteem and volunteering among older adults requires further study in the future.

Nevertheless, we found that older adults with increased self-esteem rather than increased self-efficacy from the volunteer program that began before COVID-19 were more likely to help neighbors/friends purchase daily necessities during the pandemic. Negative social media message about COVID-19 has portrayed the older population as vulnerable, helpless, and expendable individuals (Soto-perez-de-celis, 2020). As self-esteem is defined as the overall evaluation of individuals' own worth, recognition of their own values and strengths (Rosenberg, 1965), the increased self-esteem could be a more critical psychological resource than increased self-efficacy among older adults to contribute to society at such critical time.

This study has several limitations. First, our sample may be subject to self-selection bias since participants were not chosen randomly. It is possible that participants in our volunteer program were more motivated to begin with. In addition, our sample was convenient data and the sample size was relatively small. Thus, the study's findings may not be generalized to general older populations. Second, we could not test the direction of the associations. Hence, it is unclear whether volunteering led to fewer depression and anxiety symptoms, or whether better mental health prompted older adults to volunteer. Likewise, we used a cross-sectional design which limited our ability to explore the casual relationship between self-esteem and volunteering during COVID-19 although Thoits and Hewitt (2001) have suggested there is a reciprocal relationship between self-esteem and volunteerism. Last, we did not have data on the incomes and social support of older adults which could be confounding variables.

Nevertheless, our findings have important practical implications. First, since the outbreak of COVID-19, older adults have been portrayed extremely unfavorably as a homogeneous and vulnerable group in public announcements and on social media (Ayalon et al., 2020). Such negative framing toward older adults ignores the fact that some of them undertake voluntary work and act as crucial element of civil society fighting the virus. Our study suggests that the influence of older adults who are capable and willing to contribute should not be overlooked during COVID-19. Second, our findings support the suggestion that promoting volunteering may be a feasible strategy for maintaining mental health during a public health crisis. NGOs and social workers can engage older adults who are capable and willing to safely contribute in helping their communities and others in need during a public health crisis. Third, despite the epidemic, we need to provide older people opportunity to contribute to their society through pro-social behaviors, at the same time maintaining social and physical distancing. However, civil society and elderly services providers need to pay attention to equity in organizing these activities, by providing more support (e.g., more education, skill training, and social support) for older adult volunteers with low levels of individual and social resources, and mingling older adult with different levels of resources in delivering volunteering activities. Finally, regular volunteering programs enhancing self-esteem among older adults should be emphasized as it is one of the key psychological resources to drive people to volunteer and their beneficial effects may be maintained even during the pandemic.

Conclusion

The outbreak of COVID-19 was a radical disruptor to older adults' lives. Yet, our study showed that some older adults still actively contributed to their communities by engaging in different types of volunteering activities during COVID-19. Our findings indicate how volunteering during COVID-19 was associated with lower severity of depression and anxiety symptoms, and older adults with increased self-esteem were more likely to volunteer in the context of COVID-19. Social workers are encouraged to engage older adults in volunteering activities on a regular and active basis to offset the risk of depression and anxiety symptoms in times of crisis with strict health and safety measures.

Data availability statement

No additional unpublished data to share.

Ethical standards

This study was approved by the Human Research Ethics Committee (HREC) of the University of Hong Kong (HREC's reference number: EA1510033).

Funding

This work was supported by The Hong Kong Jockey Club Charities Trust under Jockey Club Age-friendly City Project (Second Phase) - Baseline Assessments, Training, District Engagement and Professional Support for Three Districts [Number: AR160070] and Research Grants Council, University Grants Committee [General Research Fund Project Number: 17614820].

ORCID

Wai Chan http://orcid.org/0000-0001-7762-221X
Cheryl Hiu Kwan Chui http://orcid.org/0000-0002-3284-5724
Johnson Chun Sing Cheung http://orcid.org/0000-0002-7837-282X
Terry Yat Sang Lum http://orcid.org/0000-0003-1196-5345
Shiyu Lu http://orcid.org/0000-0002-9355-4883

References

Afolabi, O. A. (2014). Do self esteem and family relations predict prosocial behaviour and social adjustment of fresh students? *Higher Education of Social Science*, 7(1), 26–34. https://doi.org/10.3968/5127

Afolabi, O. A., & Alade, M. O. (2015). Self efficacy and locus of control as predictors of prosocial behaviour and organizational commitment among a sample of Nigerian nurses. *Nigerian Journal of Psychology*, 20(1), 214–227.

Allen, N. J., & Rushton, J. P. (1983). Personality characteristics of community mental health volunteers: A review. *Journal of Voluntary Action Research*, 12(1), 36–49. https://doi.org/10.1177/089976408301200106

Ayalon, L., Chasteen, A., Diehl, M., Levy, B. R., Neupert, S. D., Rothermund, K., Tesch-Römer, C., & Wahl, H.-W. (2020). Aging in times of the COVID-19 pandemic: Avoiding ageism and fostering intergenerational solidarity. *The Journals of Gerontology: Series B*, 76(2), e49-e52. https://doi.org/10.1093/geronb/gbaa051

Bandura, A. (1977). Self-efficacy - toward a unifying theory of behavioral change. *Psychological Review*, 84(2), 191–215. https://doi.org/10.1037/0033-295x.84.2.191

Bonanad, C., García-Blas, S., Tarazona-Santabalbina, F., Sanchis, J., Bertomeu-González, V., Fácila, L., Ariza, A., Núñez, J., & Cordero, A. (2020). The effect of age on mortality in patients with COVID-19: A meta-analysis with 611,583 subjects. *Journal of the American Medical Directors Association*, 21(7), 915–918. https://doi.org/10.1016/j.jamda.2020.05.045

Burr, J. A., Han, S. H., & Tavares, J. L. (2015). Volunteering and cardiovascular disease risk: Does helping others get "Under the Skin?". *The Gerontologist*, 56(5), 937–947. https://doi.org/10.1093/geront/gnv032

Chambré, S. M. (1993). Volunteerism by elders: Past trends and future prospects. *The Gerontologist*, 33(2), 221–229. https://doi.org/10.1093/geront/33.2.221

Cheng, S.-T., & Hamid, P. N. (1995). An error in the use of translated scales: The Rosenberg Self-Esteem Scale for Chinese. *Perceptual and Motor Skills*, *81*(2), 431–434. https://doi.org/10.1177/003151259508100214

Choi, N. G., & Kim, J. (2011). The effect of time volunteering and charitable donations in later life on psychological wellbeing. *Ageing and Society*, *31*(4), 590–610. https://doi.org/10.1017/S0144686X10001224

Drewelies, J., Wagner, J., Tesch-Römer, C., Heckhausen, J., & Gerstorf, D. (2017). Perceived control across the second half of life: The role of physical health and social integration. *Psychology and Aging*, *32*(1), 76–92. https://doi.org/10.1037/pag0000143

Filges, T., Siren, A., Fridberg, T., & Nielsen, B. C. V. (2020). Voluntary work for the physical and mental health of older volunteers: A systematic review [10.1002/cl2.1124]. *Campbell Systematic Reviews*, *16*(4), e1124. https://doi.org/10.1002/cl2.1124

Fletcher, D., MacKenzie, D., & Villouta, E. (2005). Modelling skewed data with many zeros: A simple approach combining ordinary and logistic regression. *Environmental and Ecological Statistics*, *12*(1), 45–54. https://doi.org/10.1007/s10651-005-6817-1

Holmes, E. A., O'Connor, R. C., Perry, V. H., Tracey, I., Wessely, S., Arseneault, L., Ballard, C., Christensen, H., Cohen Silver, R., Everall, I., Ford, T., John, A., Kabir, T., King, K., Madan, I., Michie, S., Przybylski, A. K., Shafran, R., Sweeney, A., Worthman, C. M., . . . Bullmore, E. (2020). Multidisciplinary research priorities for the COVID-19 pandemic: A call for action for mental health science. *The Lancet Psychiatry*, *7*(6), 547–560. https://doi.org/10.1016/S2215-0366(20)30168-1

Jiang, D., Warner, L. M., Chong, A. M., Li, T., Wolff, J. K., & Chou, K. L. (2020). Promoting volunteering among older adults in Hong Kong: A Randomized Controlled Trial. *The Gerontologist*, *60*(5), 968–977. https://doi.org/10.1093/geront/gnz076

Lum, T. Y., & Lightfoot, E. (2005). The effects of volunteering on the physical and mental health of older people. *Research on Aging*, *27*(1), 31–55. https://doi.org/10.1177/0164027504271349

Mak, H. W., & Fancourt, D. (2020). Predictors of engaging in voluntary work during the Covid-19 pandemic: Analyses of data from 31,890 adults in the UK.

Manning, W. G., Basu, A., & Mullahy, J. (2005). Generalized modeling approaches to risk adjustment of skewed outcomes data. *Journal of Health Economics*, *24*(3), 465–488. https://doi.org/10.1016/j.jhealeco.2004.09.011

Morrow-Howell, N. (2010). Volunteering in later life: Research frontiers. *The Journals of Gerontology: Series B*, *65B*(4), 461–469. https://doi.org/10.1093/geronb/gbq024

Morrow-Howell, N., Hinterlong, J., & Sherraden, M. (2001). *Productive aging: Concepts and challenges*. Johns Hopkins University Press.

Niebuur, J., van Lente, L., Liefbroer, A. C., Steverink, N., & Smidt, N. (2018). Determinants of participation in voluntary work: A systematic review and meta-analysis of longitudinal cohort studies. *Bmc Public Health*, *18*(1), 1213. https://doi.org/10.1186/s12889-018-6077-2

Rosenberg, M. (1965). *Society and the adolescent self-image*. Princeton University Press.

Russell, A. R., Nyame-Mensah, A., de Wit, A., & Handy, F. (2019). Volunteering and wellbeing among ageing adults: A longitudinal analysis. *VOLUNTAS: International Journal of Voluntary and Nonprofit Organizations*, *30*(1), 115–128. https://doi.org/10.1007/s11266-018-0041-8

Ryon, H. S., & Gleason, M. E. J. (2014). The role of locus of control in daily life. *Personality & Social Psychology Bulletin*, *40*(1), 121–131. https://doi.org/10.1177/0146167213507087

Santini, Z. I., Jose, P. E., York Cornwell, E., Koyanagi, A., Nielsen, L., Hinrichsen, C., Meilstrup, C., Madsen, K. R., & Koushede, V. (2020). Social disconnectedness, perceived isolation, and symptoms of depression and anxiety among older Americans (NSHAP):

A longitudinal mediation analysis. *The Lancet Public Health, 5*(1), e62–e70. https://doi.org/10.1016/S2468-2667(19)30230-0

Schulz, R., & Heckhausen, J. (1999). Aging, culture and control: Setting a new research agenda. *Journals of Gerontology Series B-Psychological Sciences and Social Sciences, 54*(3), P139–145P. https://doi.org/10.1093/geronb/54B.3.P139

Sin, N. L., Klaiber, P., Wen, J. H., & DeLongis, A. (2020). Helping amid the pandemic: Daily affective and social implications of COVID-19-related prosocial activities. *The Gerontologist, 61*(1), 59–70. https://doi.org/10.1093/geront/gnaa140

Smith, M. L., Steinman, L. E., & Casey, E. A. (2020). Combatting social isolation among older adults in a time of physical distancing: The COVID-19 social connectivity paradox. *Perspective, 8*(403). https://doi.org/10.3389/fpubh.2020.00403

Soto-perez-de-celis, E. (2020). Social media, ageism, and older adults during the COVID-19 pandemic. *EClinicalMedicine, 29–30*, 100634. https://doi.org/10.1016/j.eclinm.2020.100634

Tang, F. Y., Morrow-Howell, N., & Hong, S. (2009). Inclusion of diverse older populations in volunteering the importance of institutional facilitation. *Nonprofit and Voluntary Sector Quarterly, 38*(5), 810–827. https://doi.org/10.1177/0899764008320195

Taniguchi, H. (2012). The determinants of formal and informal volunteering: Evidence from the American time use survey. *Voluntas: International Journal of Voluntary and Nonprofit Organizations, 23*(4), 920–939. https://doi.org/10.1007/s11266-011-9236-y

Thoits, P. A., & Hewitt, L. N. (2001). Volunteer work and well-being. *Journal of Health and Social Behavior, 42*(2), 115–131. https://doi.org/10.2307/3090173

Tong, X., An, D., McGonigal, A., Park, S.-P., & Zhou, D. (2016). Validation of the generalized anxiety disorder-7 (GAD-7) among Chinese people with epilepsy. *Epilepsy Research, 120*, 31–36. https://doi.org/10.1016/j.eplepsyres.2015.11.019

United Nations. (2020). *Policy brief: COVID-19 and the need for action on mental health.* Available at: https://www.un.org/sites/un2.un.org/files/un_policy_brief-covid_and_mental_health_final.pdf

Wan, K. M., Ho, L. K. K., Wong, N. W. M., & Chiu, A. (2020). Fighting COVID-19 in Hong Kong: The effects of community and social mobilization. *World Development, 134*, 105055. https://doi.org/10.1016/j.worlddev.2020.105055

Wu, Z. S., Zhao, R., Zhang, X. L., & Liu, F. Q. (2018). The impact of social capital on volunteering and giving: Evidence From Urban China. *Nonprofit and Voluntary Sector Quarterly, 47*(6), 1201–1222. https://doi.org/10.1177/0899764018784761

Yeung, A., Fung, F., Yu, S. C., Vorono, S., Ly, M., Wu, S., & Fava, M. (2008). Validation of the Patient Health Questionnaire-9 for depression screening among Chinese Americans. *Comprehensive Psychiatry, 49*(2), 211–217. https://doi.org/10.1016/j.comppsych.2006.06.002

Zhang, J. X., & Schwarzer, R. (1995). Measuring optimistic self-beliefs: A Chinese adaptation of the General Self-Efficacy Scale. *Psychologia: An International Journal of Psychology in the Orient, 38*(3), 174–181. https://psycnet.apa.org/record/1996-35921-001

Exploring the Impact of COVID-19 Pandemic on Economic Activities and Well-being of Older Adults in South-eastern Nigeria: Lessons for Gerontological Social Workers

Patricia Uju Agbawodikeizu (iD), Chigozie Donatus Ezulike (iD),
Prince Chiagozie Ekoh (iD), Elizabeth Onyedikachi George (iD),
Uzoma Odera Okoye (iD) and Ikechukwu Nnebe

ABSTRACT

The novel COVID-19 pandemic and its containment measures such as lockdown and physical distancing are remarkably affecting older adults' economic activities and well-being in ways deserving of urgent attention. To strengthen caregiving and promote targeted care for older adults during and after the pandemic, this paper investigates the impact of the coronavirus on the economic activities and well-being of older adults in Enugu and Anambra states, Nigeria. Hermeneutic phenomenology was adopted and 16 older adults aged between 60 and 81 years, with a majority of them still working as farmers and traders were phone-interviewed. Findings highlighted four key lessons for gerontological social workers including 1) the fear that impact of the containment measures could kill the older adults faster than the virus; 2) the measures generate a feeling of neglect and marginalization of healthcare needs among older adults; 3) altered positive health-seeking behavior among the older adults; 4) and concern about the absence of functional policy and plan to address the welfare of older adults. Therefore, the central focus of the gerontological social workers and Nigerian polity should not be on how to reduce the spread of the disease alone, but on an application of caution in instituting and implementing the measures.

Introduction

The coronavirus pandemic has different impacts on diverse socio-demographic groups. Specifically, it is having a more telling effect on older adults in ways deserving of urgent attention as they are reported to be more affected than other age groups worldwide (Lee, 2020; Sandoiu, 2020). This is because the health profile of older adults is characterized by limiting health conditions (Jaul & Barron, 2017), decreased immunity, comorbidity, chronic illnesses, declining physical functions and impaired socialization necessitating

increased demand on healthcare services (Olagundoye et al., 2020); consequently, it has the potential of increasing their risk of COVID-19 infection and
death. The World Health Organization [WHO] (2020) revealed that over 95%
of COVID-19 deaths worldwide occur among individuals above 60 years of
age, with over half of these deaths occurring in people aged 80 years and over.

The COVID-19 pandemic has exacerbated the needs of older people in
Nigeria, who have been shown to be in need of care and protection including
medical, financial, social and emotional support (Olagundoye et al., 2020). The
pandemic has also increased marginalization of the older adults due to the
focusing of health resources on COVID-19, thus creating barriers in their
access to healthcare services and treatment of underlying conditions (United
Nations [UN], 2020). Contrary to findings in the studies conducted in
Western countries, early research evidence in Nigeria shows the limited health
impact of the pandemic on older people and pointed to an age group spanning
21–44 years as the population with the highest infection and mortality rate
(Ajisegiri et al., 2020; Hassan et al., 2020; Nigeria Centre for Disease Control,
2020). Given the cumulative record of infection rate of the virus, the Nigerian
government has instituted measures to control its widespread, and such
measures include physical distancing, avoidance of social and religious gatherings, lockdowns, and self-isolation (Olagundoye et al., 2020). These measures
may adversely affect the well-being, social engagements, contacts and financial
support of older adults and their caregiving arrangements (Brooke & Jackson,
2020; Olagundoye et al., 2020).

The COVID-19 pandemic is also affecting the older adults economically.
Although it is stereotypical for older people in Nigeria perceived as to be
retirees, older persons who retire from civil service, and are still active, often
engage in income-earning activities such as farming and petty trading to
augment the very limited pension scheme (Apere, 2015; Daramola et al.,
2018; Garba & Usman, 2014) while those who did not work in civil service
and thus received no pensions also engage in farming and petty trading to earn
a livelihood, and as well depend on the support from family and friends
(Daramola et al., 2018). The economic status of these groups of older adults
may likely be adversely affected due to the economic crisis orchestrated by the
pandemic. The UN (2020) notes that the aging population experience challenges in meeting most of their essential needs given the lockdown, increased
living costs and closure of economic activities. Also noted in the UN (2020)
report is the threat the pandemic poses to older adults' jobs, pension and
mental health given that those who receive care at home and in the community
are at risk of being disproportionately affected by physical distancing measures. This could affect the amount of support family members avail their
older kin. Nigeria is the first Sub-Saharan African country to record the index
case of COVID-19 (WHO, 2020) and the pandemic is already overwhelming
the nation's economic capacity required to strengthen the health systems for

containment of its widespread as well as provide adequate support to the populace to reduce its effects (United Nation Development Program [UNDP], 020). Additionally, with the unprecedented increase in the population of Nigerian older adults which was put at 9.3 million in 2019, and the dependency ratio of 5 older adults per 100 persons aged 15–59 (United Nations Department of Economic and Social Affairs, Population Division, 2019; Olagundoye et al., 2020) there is no functional national policy (Tanyi et al., 2018) nor social welfare program to address their care and welfare. This includes the lack of unemployment compensation and little or no disaster relief to cope with the economic hardship of the pandemic (Arthur-Holmes et al., 2020; Ozili, 2020). Similarly, the very limited pension schemes which provides limited income and covers only older adults who are retirees (Fapohunda, 2013), are highly suggestive of the plight of older adults reflected in a further decline in their economic situation during the COVID-19 pandemic. Therefore, exploring the impacts of COVID-19 pandemic on the economic activities and well-being of Nigeria's older persons is necessary and timely.

Some studies in the United States have assessed the impact of COVID-19 pandemic on the economic condition and well-being of older adults and reported that the pandemic worsens the economic situation, health and well-being of older persons. For instance, Pestine-Stevens and Greenfield (2020), and Yang and Jan (2020), highlighted in their findings that the impact of the COVID-19 crisis may worsen the economic condition for many Americans aged 65 years or older, especially those who live in places where high infection rates and high economic risks occur, and those with fewer sources and lower levels of income, given that some of them lose wages and others exhaust their savings to weather the economic downturn. Morrow-Howell et al. (2020) in their review reported that the closing of organizations and self-isolation orders due to COVID-19 crisis has prevented many older persons from having their preexisting physical, emotional and social needs met. The authors further noted that the healthcare system has narrowed its focus to managing COVID-19 cases thereby delaying other healthcare appointments (such as regular checkups) and putting older patients at high risk of worsening health deterioration.

On the other hand, the few studies that investigated the impact of the pandemic in Nigeria zoomed in on how COVID-19 has affected the nation and some vulnerable groups, specifically younger people. The United Nations High Commissioner for Refugees [UNHCR] (2020) assessed the impact of the pandemic on persons of concern in Nigeria and reported that COVID-19 affected several vulnerable groups (Refugees, Internally Displaced Persons [IDPs], and returnees) with most of them experiencing reduced income and loss of income as a result of restrictive measures imposed by the government. Also, the UNDP (2020) in their assessment of the impact of the pandemic reported that the health crisis has adverse effects on the overall economic activities in the country including domestic trade and services which account for the bulk of the GDP. However, none of these studies in Nigeria focused on assessing the impact of COVID-19 on older people considering that they are classified as a vulnerable population (National Primary Health Care Development Agency, 2020; WHO, 2020). This study, therefore, aimed to identify lessons that will be key in strengthening caregiving and promoting targeted care for older adults through the wake and after the pandemic by qualitatively exploring the impact of the coronavirus pandemic on the economic activities and well-being of older adults in Enugu and Anambra states, Nigeria.

We further adopted the political economy theory of aging in explaining the economic situation of aged persons during the COVID-19 pandemic. The main premise of the theory is that poverty in old age is a function of the low economic and social status of the aged population before and after retirement, and secondly, of the relatively low level of state benefits (Alan, 2008). The theorist argues that social policies which have failed to recognize inequality in old age and the causes of low economic and social status among the elderly have therefore failed to tackle the problem of poverty and low income of the aged population. Thus, how economic challenge among older people is defined and the type of remedy provided to address it reflect how the government (social policies) perceives the old (Estes et al., 1996). Nigeria is not a welfare state, as aged care is perceived to be a family responsibility (Tanyi et al., 2018). Hence, in the era of COVID-19 pandemic, older persons are bound to face economic challenges, including poverty. Being helping professionals, social workers in aged care focus their research interest on older adults' caregiving issues. Although Onalu et al. (2020) noted that the training provided to social workers in Nigeria is inadequate to inform a response to health emergencies because they lacked awareness of the roles expected of them in response to the pandemic following their training curriculum, findings from our study, therefore, have lessons for social workers in aged care with a focus on strengthening caregiving and promoting targeted care to older adults. The questions that guided the study include: What are the impacts of the coronavirus pandemic on older adults and how does it affect the economic activities and well-being of older adults in Enugu and Anambra states, Nigeria?

Materials and methods

The dire impact of COVID-19 pandemic on the economic activities and well-being of a significant number of older adults in Nigeria is a reflection of their poverty level, low economic status, and the access they have to the resources for health. The precepts of the political economy theory were essential in the approach we adopted in this study. This is because a great deal of research on aging in Nigeria stereotyped and treated the older persons as a homogenous group with special needs (Ajayi et al., 2015; Fapohunda, 2013; Hassan et al., 2020; Olagundoye et al., 2020; Tanyi et al., 2018), and little attention has been paid to the impact of public health emergencies on their individual lived experiences. We, therefore, adopted the Hermeneutic phenomenology for this study due to its suitability in exploring individuals' lived experience of a phenomenon (Manen, 2018). Hermeneutic phenomenology focuses on investigating and making meaning of participants' lived experiences from their perspectives and interpretations (Manen, 2018). We followed this research tradition because of its fit in describing and interpreting a phenomenon, which in this case is, the impact of COVID-19 on the economic activities and wellbeing of older adults. A study designed to explore the impact of COVID-19 on economic activities and wellbeing of older adults from the perspectives and experiences of the older adults themselves lends itself to phenomenological research.

The study was carried out in Enugu and Anambra states due to the notable economic activities carried out therein (Agu, 2016). Enugu and Anambra are among the five states that make up the Southeast geopolitical zone in Nigeria. The states are predominantly characterized by their economic activities such as trading and farming (Agu, 2016); of which older residents in the states, including those who are retirees, still engage in to earn a living and support their pension.

Non-probability sampling methods such as purposive, availability and snowball sampling were adopted in selecting 16 older persons who were aged between 60 and 81 years: eight each from the states. A sample size of 16 is suitable for a qualitative study such as phenomenology as it allows for variation and saturation of quality narratives of individuals' lived experiences (Creswell, 2006). To select the study participants, two of the researchers, one each from the two states liaised with a few family relations/caregivers of older persons (who are well known to them) who served to assist in recruiting the older persons residing with them. The researchers asked the relatives/care-givers to speak to the older people about the study and find out if they were interested in participating, and then, communicate the response to the researchers through the contact information exchanged. The caregivers gave the researchers the phone numbers of older persons who agreed to participate in the study and were comfortable with the data collection method. These older persons were then used to sample other participants within their reach. A total of 24 older people were reached out to, however, only 16 were: willing to participate in the study. Criteria for inclusion in the study include engaging in trading/or farming as a major source of livelihood or having retired from the civil service, and being able/willing to engage in a telephone conversation for up to a maximum of 60 minutes. We included older adults who engaged in income-earning activities such as farming and/or trading and the retirees due to the focus of the study. Our choice was also informed by the predominant occupation of the older adults who were contacted and recruited for the study and a significant number of the retirees who also engage in farming and petty trading.

The study was carried out at a time when the states were on lockdown with the instituted travel ban, and we considered a physically distant approach more appropriate. Thus, a telephone interview was adopted as the method of data collection to minimize the risks of exposing older persons to the COVID-19 virus which spreads mostly through close contact with an infected person (WHO, 2020). Although telephone interviews are considered inferior by many qualitative researchers and may pose some constraints due to service connectivity issues, electronic qualitative tools are emerging relevant data collection methods (Drabble et al., 2016), especially considering the need to stay safe while conducting the study. The interviews were conducted by two of the researchers from these states who understand the language and are trained researchers and social workers. Before commencing the interviews, the researchers established a good rapport with the respondents via phone calls. The respondents were assured of the anonymity of their identities, and they gave their consent verbally, and selected convenient dates and time for the interviews. During the interviews, each participant's consent was verbally obtained before we commenced recording of the conversation, and we used Android phones with the call-recording feature for the recording. Each of the interviews lasted for an average of 58 minutes and were conducted in the respondents' local dialects which are also the local dialects of the two interviewers. Expressions like 'hmmm', 'okay', 'yes?', 'really', 'ndo' (meaning sorry) were used to convey listening.

Data collection lasted for 5 weeks; from mid-April to mid-May, 2020. The audio files were transcribed verbatim in the local dialects and translated to English (by the two researchers who conducted the interviews and two other researchers who understand the language). Data analysis was done thematically and in line with hermeneutic phenomenological research principles, namely: reflection, immersion, and categorization. The transcripts were given to all the researchers who did manual coding by getting immersed in the text and seeing what common themes flowed from the transcripts. We reflected on the interviewees' narratives by conducting multiple reads of both individual transcripts and the entire interview as a single text to make meaning of their shared experiences and interpretations. After the multiple reads of the transcripts, each of the authors made notes of identified emerging ideas which were then categorized into themes. All researchers switched notes to double-check for quality assurance and drew comprehensive central themes for the discussion. Themes that were identified by one author but not others were discussed and debated based on the transcripts, and either accepted or discarded depending on the evidence other authors saw or did not see from the research. This helped with the trustworthiness of the study as it made it difficult for the results to be influenced by the biases and interpretations of any single author. To further enhance the trustworthiness of this study, we: selected participants who met the requirements for the study and could articulate their experiences; conducted the interviews in language the participants were comfortable with and could easily understand; chose to conduct the study in settings we are largely familiar with to reduce the chances of important information being lost in translation; critically assessed one another's inputs, and provided a detailed description of the study participants and settings in case transferability is considered.

Before the interviews, the participants were duly informed about the purpose of the study, how they were selected, what would be done with the data, their right to decline participation or responding to any questions, and the confidentiality of information shared. Ethical approval for this study was granted by the Research Ethics Review Board of the Department of Psychology, University of Nigeria Nsukka (ref: PSY/REC/UNN/20/IRB-0000-030).

Results

Social demographics of the respondents

A total of 16 respondents were recruited from the two study sites, eight of them were from Enugu while the other eight were from Anambra. Nine of the respondents were females and six were males. The age distribution of the respondents shows that five were aged between 60 and 69, 10 were aged between 70 and 79, and only one was 81 years old. Eight of the respondents were traders, two were farmers and six were retired. The respondents' level of education shows that eight of them had primary education, six had no formal education while two had secondary education. Seven of the respondents lived with their children, five lived with their children and spouses and four lived alone.

Three major themes were identified from the narratives of the respondents' lived experiences. The major themes reflect the impact of the pandemic containment measures and how they affect different facets of economic activities and the well-being of older adults, as well as the perceived support from the government. Table 1 captures the major themes and associated sub-themes that emerged from the data analysis.

Table 1. Major themes and sub-themes from the data analysis.

Major themes	Sub-themes
Impact of the lockdown order on economic activities of the older adults	Difficulty in feeding (hunger) and reduced standard of living orchestrated by movement restrictions
Impact on well-being	Increased difficulties in assessing health care services among older adults
Support from the government	Sporadic and highly limited support from the government

Source: *Data collected on impact of COVID-19 on older adults in Nigeria, 2020.*

Impact of the lockdown order on economic activities of the older adults

The lockdown order instituted by the government to contain the widespread of the coronavirus was identified as major distress to the viable economic and income-generating activities engaged in by the respondents. The majority of those who engaged in poultry farming and sale of beverages recounted their losses including an increased death rate of their birds, high cost of feed and drugs, reduced productivity, and poor sale of "drinks" due to restrictions on public gatherings, among others. Also, one of the respondents pointed out that her children no longer send foodstuffs to her due to movement restrictions and that she has no fear of dying of COVID-19 but hunger due to lack of food. The impacts as experienced and expressed by the respondents from Ihe (a community in Enugu state) are illustrated with the following quotes:

> Yes, this poultry I'm doing, it affected it o. Most of my fowls died. And their feed is very costly and their drugs became too costly. It made me reduce the rate at which I feed them which made them reduce productivity. (P2- Female, 68, Farmer).

> How it affected me is that things are not moving well again. Business is not moving especially for us that sell drinks. Something like burials or wedding ceremonies, they don't do that again and from it we make sales. Ever since when the lockdown started, it has affected our business. (P3- Male, 72, Trader).

> My children used to bring food to me but not anymore. My son, who will help me? I don't go to the farm again due to my ill-health and I don't go to the market to buy things. As for me, I am not afraid of the coronavirus killing me but the hunger that the lockdown brought upon me. (P5- Female, 79, Retiree).

In addition to the narratives from Ihe, some of the respondents from Aroma, Awka, a community in Anambra state indicated that the impact of the pandemic was felt differently according to people's finance and sustaining capacity. Also mentioned was a belief that the lockdown was used to punish the citizens as they were mandated to sit at home with no support from the government, and that hunger, orchestrated by the lockdown, kills the older adults faster than the coronavirus. One of the respondents noted as follows:

> The essence is to stop the spread of coronavirus but it was used to punish the population with hunger. For instance, we traders can only eat if we go to the shop to sell. With

lockdown, people were forced to sit at home without aid from the government. It is only a few people who brought noodles but they are not enough. Some families were able to get two packs or more. People suffered and are still suffering on the account of lockdown by the government. They said we should not come out of our homes to avoid us contracting COVID-19 and dying of it but hunger caused by this lockdown is even fast killing us than the virus. (P10- Female, 68, Trader).

Further, the respondents continued to illustrate how the pandemic impacts their economic activities by mentioning that they lacked financial support, their monthly income dropped since the lockdown period and cost of living is high.

Difficulty in feeding (hunger) and reduced standard of living orchestrated by movement restrictions

Also, within the context of the impact of the pandemic on economic activities, the respondents indicated that the lockdown made foodstuff to be expensive with no money to purchase the food items. It equally affected their feeding as they feed less, ration food and manage to stay alive. It affected the support given to them by their children and other relatives and engendered hunger which they continued to fear that it could kill them faster than the virus. The experiences of the respondents as expressed are illustrated with the following quotes: "Yes, it is true because feeding is now difficult in this lockdown due to the economic situation of the country. I even fear so many of us will die of hunger before we contract the coronavirus sef" (P13- Male, 65, Aroma, Trader). "Yes, it affected my feeding immensely as we now ration food to ensure there will be some to keep body and soul together tomorrow, not necessarily eating to enjoy or get filled up" (P6- Male, 73, Aroma, Retired).

Another concern expressed by one of the respondents is phrased as follows:

Coronavirus affected my feeding so bad that my children find it difficult to provide for me. My children and some other family members don't assist me as they used to because of the physical distancing order by the government. While they insist that I do not go out but lock myself indoors to stay safe from catching the virus, they do not know that hunger may kill me soon in the absence of support with food (P10, Female, 68, Aroma, Trader).

Impact on well-being

Increased difficulties in accessing health care services among older adults

Added to the recounts on impact encountered on the economic activities of the older adults are impacts on their well-being. Older adults have encountered difficulties receiving medical services at health facilities due to the focus of health resources on COVID-19 and the physical distancing and lockdown measures. This stalled their routine checkup, and thus creating barriers to their access to health-care services. They felt neglected and their access to health-care services is marginalized. Also, those who did not want to use the health facilities feared testing positive to COVID-19 and being forced to quarantine and be branded a COVID-19 patient. In the respondents' views: "Yes, it's affecting my health. If we are not asked to stay at home and maintain physical and social distancing, my children would have been coming around to take me to the hospital for a checkup" (P4- Female, 81, Ihe, Retired). "Visiting the hospital currently is also a challenge as many of us feared being told that we are or tested positive to COVID-19 and being held in isolation or be quarantined and mistaken or even termed COVID-19 patients" (P6- Male, 73, Aroma, Retired). Other concerns as expressed by a respondent include:

> Yes, it affects us the elderly more, receiving medical attention in the hospitals these days is difficult, you'll be asked to cover the nose and mouth before anyone can attend to you. The nurses will be avoiding you like you already have the disease and sometimes, no one will attend to you, you just wait and when you are tired of waiting to be attended to, you will go back to your home (P7- Female, 75, Aroma, Trader).

Also highlighted was that the affected income status of the older adults made them unable to purchase their routine drugs for their ill health: "It affected it. I can no longer afford to buy all the drugs for myself. I need drugs for my BP, waist pain and arthritis but I can no longer afford to buy the drugs" (P14- Male, 78, Aroma, Trader).

Support from the government

Sporadic and highly limited support from the government

Responses on support from the government reveal that the government has been perceived as not having any plan for the welfare of the aging population. The government occasionally shared foodstuff (rice and yam); though it was inadequate, and even the retirees have to beg to receive their pensions, which do not come regularly. Opinions of the respondents are phrased in the following quotes: "I have not noticed any government intervention. In my opinion, the government is not doing anything relating to our wellbeing in this country, I have to be honest to you" (P10- Female, 68, Aroma, Trader). "Only what they did was to share us rice and yam just once, and these items were not enough and didn't last for me" (P1- Male, 72, Ihe, Retired). Added views from other respondents are illustrated as follows:

> The government does not have any plan for the elders in this country even some of us that worked for the government have to beg to receive our pensions which does not come regularly. Like now, they shared noodles to us which is not right because we old ones should not eat that, it is meant for children. What we eat is something like rice, yam, garri, etc that can help sustain us (P9- Male, 73, Ihe, Retired).

In their suggestions, the respondents noted that the government should distribute medicines (consumables) as incentives to the older adults in rural areas and that the distribution should be done in a way that it will reach directly to the designated and not through third parties. The need for the government to apply caution in instituting/adopting measures to control the widespread of the virus was highlighted as some of the measures may cause more harm to the people than the virus. Suggestions of the respondents are presented as follows:

> Distributing medicines and medical equipment to the elderly will go a long way mostly to those in rural areas and do not have anyone to take care or provide for them even if it is just vitamin C and some incentives to keep body and soul together. I will also suggest the government should distribute the incentives in a way it will get to the designated directly and not through third parties (P8- Female, 78, Aroma Community, Retired).

> The government needs to be cautious about methods they use and those they still plan to use in future to control the spread of the disease because some of the methods may cause more harm to the people than the virus itself (P16- Female, 73, Ihe, Farmer).

Discussion

This paper reported that due to the lockdown, restrictions on freedom of movement and physical distancing measures in response to the COVID-19 pandemic, older adults who engaged in economic and income yielding activities recorded losses in their business ventures, reduced productivity, had no financial support from their family and the government, and had a huge drop in their monthly income. They equally experienced an increase in the cost of living, reduced purchasing power, and reduced living standards. These affected their feeding and engendered poverty and hunger among them, thus triggering in them, a feeling of fear that hunger could kill them even faster than the coronavirus. This means that while the health systems' the government's and organizations' COVID-19 response plans target containment of the health crisis and protection of the masses through the instituted measures, little/no emphasis was laid on putting in place social support measures to address the consequence of the infection containment measures on the older adults in particular given that they are the most affected age group. As a result, the pandemic's containment measures were highlighted to have a hard hit on the economic activities and well-being of older adults. The findings of this study were highlighted in the reports of other similar studies (Arthur-Holmes et al., 2020; Yang and Jan, 2020; Ozili, 2020; UN, 2020) which noted the challenges experienced by the aged population due to the lockdown, including low economic status reflected in their inability to meet most of their essential needs, increased living costs, closure of economic activities, loss of jobs, loss of wages, overwhelming of their savings, among others.

Findings from this study revealed that the older adults encountered diffi-culty accessing and utilizing medical services at health facilities due to focusing of health resources on COVID-19 and the physical distancing and lockdown measures. They felt neglected and their access to health-care services and resources marginalized. Those who did not want to use the health facilities feared testing positive to COVID-19 and being branded COVID-19 patients. This study also found that the affected income level of the older adults and its resultant reduction in their purchasing power made them unable to buy their routine drugs for their ill-health. This corroborates the reports that the emergence of the COVID-19 pandemic has necessitated increased demand for health-care services (Olagundoye et al., 2020) and focusing of health resources on COVID-19 cases (UN, 2020). The effect of overwhelming the healthcare system, therefore, could be felt by the masses, especially among the age group with limiting health conditions who will experience limited access to health services (Jaul & Barron, 2017; Olagundoye et al., 2020). Substantiating the findings of this paper, Morrow-Howell et al. (2020) highlighted that the closing of organizations, self-isolation orders, and narrowing the focus of the health-care system due to the COVID-19 crisis prevented meeting the preex-isting physical, emotional and social needs of many older people, as well as caused delays to their other health-care appointments.

This paper revealed that the government of Nigeria has been perceived by the sampled older adults as having a minimal plan for the welfare of the aging population as they provided little assistance to these individuals to cushion the effects of the pandemic, and even the retirees, for instance, have to beg to receive their pension which comes irregularly. This could be because aged care in Nigeria is largely perceived to be a family responsibility (Tanyi et al., 2018). Thus, the government may not likely consider a policy or welfare program to address the welfare needs of the older adults among its priority in the pan-demic response plan. However, given the nation's lack of a functional national policy and social welfare program to address the care and welfare of the aging population (Tanyi et al., 2018) and the lack of unemployment compensation and disaster relief to cope with the economic hardship of the pandemic (Ozili, 2020), older persons are indeed bound to face economic challenges during the COVID-19 pandemic and beyond.

Alan's (2008) political economy theory of aging provided a better under-standing of the findings of this study as the pandemic contributed to the poverty level experienced by the older adults which the theory described as a function of their low economic and social status. Another basic contribution of the theory to the study is the idea that poverty in old age is a factor of the relatively low level of state benefit. This idea was evidenced in the findings of the study as the older adults affirmed that the government provided little or no state benefit to them to ease their economic challenges, and this may be due to the absence of functional national policy in Nigeria to address the care and welfare of older adults. Further, the theory perceived poverty in old age as another determinant of older persons' access to health resources, however, findings from this study, show that in addition to poverty, the decision not to use health resources/facilities by some older adults due to fear of testing positive to COVID-19 and being branded COVID-19 patients is a considerable factor.

The field of gerontology in the social work discipline is relatively young in Nigeria, and the non-professionalization of social work limits the activities of gerontological social workers in Nigeria. Nevertheless, social workers in Nigeria still make noticeable efforts to influence policies that improve the lives of vulnerable people in the country through advocacy programs, culture-sensitive intervention programs to improve the lives of Nigerians and invest in researches aimed at informing policies. Therefore, the findings of this study highlight four key lessons for social workers in aged care with a focus on strengthening caregiving and promoting targeted care for older adults. The first is that the COVID-19 containment measures instituted by the government generated an unintended consequence (hunger) which triggered a feeling of fear among the older adults that it could kill them faster than the virus.

Second, the study highlights how focusing of health resources on COVID-19 and the physical distancing and lockdown measures generated a feeling of neglect and marginalization of healthcare needs and access to health services among the older adults. Third, the findings show how an otherwise positive health-seeking behavior among the older adults can be altered and characterized by an unwillingness to use health facilities due to fear of testing positive to COVID-19 and being held in isolation and branded COVID-19 patients. This could be as a result of the attitude of the health personnel toward the patients. The fourth is that our study found that the government has no plan for the welfare of older adults. This may explain why the COVID-19 pandemic and its containment measures adversely affect the well-being, social and financial support of older adults (Brooke & Jackson, 2020; Olagundoye et al., 2020). Accordingly, our study has evidenced that restrictions on freedom of movement and physical distancing can lead to interruption of vital care and support for older adults. Drawing on these lessons, therefore, the central focus of gerontological social workers in responding to care for older adults during pandemics is to recognize and promote that infection containment measures are important but need to be accompanied by social support measures and targeted care for the older adults.

Findings from this study have implications for policy, practice, and research. With the relatively low level of economic development in Nigeria and the expectation of the people to live and survive to old age, results from this study show that the government (both at national and sub-national levels) must design innovative policies targeted at the provision of care and social support for older adults and mitigation of effects of public health emergencies on them. This will facilitate all-inclusive planning and management of the pandemic and future outbreaks.

The four key lessons indicated in the findings of this study are presented to inform the work of gerontological social workers practicing in Nigeria. Finally, findings from this study only revealed the impacts of the COVID-19 pandemic and its containment measures on the economic activities and well-being of older adults, and this suggests the need for more research on the same phenomenon focusing on other areas of older adults'livelihood.

The main strength of this study is that it is foremost to assess the experiences of older Nigerians concerning their economic and welfare needs during the COVID-19 pandemic and document the empirical report. The limitations are the use of phone interviews, which did not allow for face-to-face interaction with the respondents, and the relatively small scale of the study, being carried out in two communities in the states, hence not allowing for comparison of situations in other communities. Further studies are also needed to assess the impact of the pandemic in other communities not investigated in this study for comparison of contexts.

The distress orchestrated by the COVID-19 pandemic on the economic activities and well-being of older adults is enormous. Disease containment measures such as the lockdown and physical distancing orders have been shown to result in disruption of care and support for older adults. Given the key lessons highlighted in the findings of this study, the question in the mind of social workers in aged care is how to advocate for and promote the incorporation of social support measures and targeted care for older adults in the disease containment measures to address the next wave of the pandemic and other pandemics in the future. In this regard, the central focus should not be how to reduce the spread of the disease, but an application of caution in instituting and implementing the disease control measures as some of the measures may cause more harm to the older adults than the virus, likewise, taking cognizance of the essence of social support and use of incentives for solidarity.

ORCID

Patricia Uju Agbawodikeizu (iD) http://orcid.org/0000-0003-1685-3449
Chigozie Donatus Ezulike (iD) http://orcid.org/0000-0002-7883-5679
Prince Chiagozie Ekoh (iD) http://orcid.org/0000-0002-1787-536X
Elizabeth Onyedikachi George (iD) http://orcid.org/0000-0001-5678-4113
Uzoma Odera Okoye (iD) http://orcid.org/0000-0002-0605-3002

References

Agu, N. N. (2016). Impacts of climate change, variability and adaptation strategies on agriculture in two agricultural communities of Enugu State, Nigeria. *International Journal of Science and Research, 5*(7), 916–921. https://doi.org/10.21275/v5i7.NOV164474

Ajayi, S. A., Adebusoye, L. A., Ogunbode, A. M., Akinyemi, J. O., & Adebayo, A. M. (2015). Profile and correlates of functional status in elderly patients presenting at a primary care clinic in Nigeria. *African Journal of Primary Health Care & Family Medicine, 7*(1), 1–7. https://doi.org/10.4102/phcfm.v7i1.810

Ajisegiri, W. S., Odusanya, O. O., & Joshi, R. (2020). COVID-19 outbreak situation in Nigeria and the need for effective engagement of community health workers for epidemic response. *Global Biosecurity, 2*(1). https://doi.org/10.31646/gbio.69

Alan, W. (2008). Towards a political economy of old age. *Ageing and Society, 1*(1), 73–94. https://doi.org/10.1017/S0144686X81000056

Apere, P. (2015). *Key challenges of Nigerian Pension Industry and possible solutions (1).* The Nation. http://thenationonlineng.net/key-challenges-of-nigerian-pension-industry-and-possible-solutions-1/

Arthur-Holmes, F., Akaadom, M. K. A., Agyemang-Duah, W., Busia, K. A., & Peprah, P. (2020). Healthcare concerns of older adults during the COVID-19 outbreak in low- and middle-income countries: Lessons for health policy and social work. *Journal of Gerontological Social Work, 63*(6–7), 717–723. https://doi.org/10.1080/01634372.2020.1800883

Brooke, J., & Jackson, D. (2020). Older people and COVID-19: Isolation, risk and ageism. *Journal of Clinical Nursing, 29*(13–14), 2044–2046. Retrieved September 29, 2020, from https://onlinelibrary.wiley.com/doi/10.1111/jocn.15274#jocn15274-bib-0004

Creswell, J. (2006). *Five qualitative approaches to inquiry.* SAGE Publications Inc. https://www.sagepub.com/sites/default/files/upm-binaries/13421_Chapter4.pdf

Daramola, O. E., Awunor, N. S., & Akande, T. M. (2018). The challenges of retirees and older persons in Nigeria; a need for close attention and urgent action. *International Journal of Tropical Disease & Health, 34*(4), 1–8. https://doi.org/10.9734/IJTDH/2018/v34i430099

Drabble, L., Trocki, K., Salcedo, B., Walker, P. C., & Korcha, R. A. (2016). Conducting qualitative interviews by telephone: Lessons learned from a study of alcohol use among sexual minority and heterosexual women. *Qualitative Social Work: Research and Practice, 15* (1), 118–133. https://doi.org/10.1177/1473325015585613

Estes, E., Linkins, K., & Binney, E. (1996). The political economy of aging. In R. Binstock & L. George (Eds.), *Handbook of aging and the social sciences* (4th ed., pp. 346–358). Academic Press.

Fapohunda, T. M. (2013). The Pension System and Retirement Planning in Nigeria. Mediterranean Journal of Social Sciences, 4(2), 25-34.

Garba, A., & Usman, H. (2014). Retirement challenges and sustainable development in Nigeria. *European Journal of Business and Management, 6*(39), 94–98. https://core.ac.uk/download/pdf/234626146.pdf

Hassan, Z., Hashim, J. M., & Khan, G. (2020). Population risk factors for COVID-19 deaths in Nigeria at sub-national level. *Pan African Medical Journal, 35*(2), 131. https://doi.org/10.11604/pamj.supp.2020.35.2.25258

Jaul, E., & Barron, J. (2017). Age-related diseases and clinical public health implications for the 85 years old and over population. *Frontiers in Public Health, 5,* 335. https://doi.org/10.3389/fpubh.2017.00335

Lee, Y. J. (2020). The impact of the COVID-19 Pandemic on vulnerable older adults in the United States. *Journal of Gerontological Social Work, 63*(6–7), 559–564. https://doi.org/10.1080/01634372.2020.1777240

Manen, M. V. (2018). *Researching lived experience* (2nd).Routledge.

Morrow-Howell, N., Galucia, N., & Swinford, E. (2020). Recovering from the COVID-19 pandemic: A focus on older adults. *Journal of Aging & Social Policy, 32*(4–5), 526–535. https://doi.org/10.1080/08959420.2020.1759758

National Primary Health Care Development Agency. (2020). *Preparedness and response to Coronavirus disease at primary healthcare and community level.* Federal Ministry of Health. https://www.humanitarianresponse.info/sites/www.humanitarianresponse.info/files/documents/files/guide_on_phc_preparedness_and_response-covid-19.pdf

Nigeria Centre for Disease Control. (2020). *COVID-19 outbreak in Nigeria situation report S/N 65.* Federal Ministry of Health. https://ncdc.gov.ng/diseases/sitreps/?cat=14&name=An%20update%20of%20COVID-19%20outbreak%20in%20Nigeria.

Olagundoye, O., Enema, O., & Adebowale, A. (2020). Recommendations for a national Coronavirus disease 2019 response guideline for the care of older persons in Nigeria during and post-pandemic: A family physician's perspective. *African Journal of Primary Health Care & Family Medicine, 12*(1), a2512. https://doi.org/10.4102/phcfm.v12i1.2512

Onalu, C. E., Chukwu, N. G., & Okoye, U. O. (2020). COVID-19 response and social work education in Nigeria: Matters arising. *Social Work Education, 39*(8), 1037–1047. https://doi.org/10.1080/02615479.2020.1825663

Ozili, P. K. (2020). COVID-19 pandemic and economic crisis: The Nigerian experience and structural causes. *Journal of Economic and Administrative Sciences.* Advance online publication. https://mpra.ub.uni-muenchen.de/103131/1/MPRA_paper_103131.pdf

Pestine-Stevens, A., & Greenfield, E. A. (2020). The need for community practice to support aging in place during COVID-19. *Journal of Gerontological Social Work, 63*(6–7), 631–634. https://doi.org/10.1080/01634372.2020.1789258

Sandoiu, A. (May 19, 2020). The impact of the COVID-19 pandemic on older adults. *Medical News Today.* Retrieved September 30, 2020, from https://www.medicalnewstoday.com/articles/the-impact-of-the-covid-19-pandemic-on-older-adults.

Tanyi, L. P., Andre, P., & Mbah, P. (2018). Care of the elderly in Nigeria: Implications for policy. *Congent Social Sciences, 4*(1), 1–14. https://doi.org/10.1080/23311886.2018.155520

United Nation Development Program. (March 24, 2020). *The impact of the COVID-19 pandemic in Nigeria: A socio-economic analysis-Brief 1.* Retrieved October 29, 2020, from https://www.ng.undp.org/content/nigeria/en/home/library/the-impact-of-the-covid-19-pandemic-in-nigeria--a-socio-economic.html.

United Nations. (2020). *Policy brief: The impact of COVID-19 on older persons.* https://unsdg.un.org/sites/default/files/2020-05/Policy-Brief-The-Impact-of-COVID-19-on-Older-Persons.pdf.

United Nations Department of Economic and Social Affairs, Population Division (2019). *World population prospects: The 2019 revision.* Accessed from: http://data.un.org/Data.aspx?d=PopDiv&f=variableID%3A67#PopDiv

United Nations High Commissioner for Refugees. (July, 2020). *Socio-economic impact assessment of COVID-19 pandemic among persons of concern in Nigeria.* Retrieved August 22, 2020, from https://reliefweb.int/report/nigeria/socio-economic-impact-assessment-covid-19-pandemic-among-persons-concern-nigeria-july

World Health Organization. (2020). *Weekly bulletin on outbreaks and other emergencies.* https://apps.who.int/iris/bitstream/handle/10665/331892/OEW17-2026042020.pdf.

Yang, L.& Jan, E. M. (2020). Older adults and the economic impact of the COVID-19 pandemic*Journal of Aging & Social Policy. 32*(4-5), 477-487. https://doi.org/10.1080/08959420.2020.1773191

Digital and Physical Social Exclusion of Older People in Rural Nigeria in the Time of COVID-19

Prince Chiagozie Ekoh(iD), Elizabeth Onyedikachi George(iD) and Chigozie Donatus Ezulike(iD)

ABSTRACT

As the use of digital technology becomes more widespread across the globe, older people remain among the group with the lowest access and usage. The digital divide may lead to double exclusion as the COVID-19 pandemic has led to limited physical social contact as experts' recommendation of continuous social distancing and lack of access and usage of internet communication will leave older people socially isolated. The aim of this study is to explore how older people in rural Nigeria may be digitally excluded and its impact during the COVID-19 pandemic. Qualitative data was obtained from 11 older people using interviews. The collected data was then transcribed and analyzed thematically. Findings show that older people in rural Nigeria were digitally excluded. However, the older people argued that the digital exclusion is not the reason for their social isolation and loneliness. The study concluded by suggesting how caregivers and social workers can assist rural older people through activity schedule and radio programs designed for older people.

Introduction

Digital technology and the internet have become major sources and resources for services, information and entertainment. Internet use influences almost all aspects of our everyday lives (Seifert, 2020; Van Deursen & Helsper, 2015). However, as internet use and access have become widespread across the globe, studies show a gap in access and usage between young people and older people (Anderson et al., 2019; Hunsaker & Hargittai, 2018). There is evidence showing that access and usage of the internet by older people have been increasing rapidly, with Office for National Statistics (2018) showing that the number of older people with access to the internet has more than doubled from 2011 to 2018. Yet people aged above 55 years make up 94% of everyone who has never used the internet (Centre for Ageing Better, 2018).

Older people are not the only social group at the lower end of this digital divide as studies have shown that there is low internet use among people with lower level of education, people with lower income, single parents, female heads of households, rural dwellers and people living in low-income countries (Anderson et al., 2019; Yang & Du, 2020). Yet older people may also fall part of this group disproportionately affected by digital exclusion, given that many older people tend to have low income, low level of education, live in rural communities, are female heads of household and living in low-income country (Roberts, 2010). Our study focuses on rural older people, with participants falling at the lower end of the digital use spectrum.

Studies have shown that factors responsible for digital exclusion of older people may include access to digital devices and internet as low income and poor internet connections in rural areas limit their access to digital technology (Formosa, 2013; Gibson et al., 2020; Mukhtar, 2020), lack of skill needed to use digital technology, and computer literacy (Blažič & Blažič, 2020; Van Bronswijk et al., 2008). For instance, Age UK (2018) reported that among people who use the internet, only 27% of those aged 65+ use social network sites like Facebook, Twitter, TikTok compared to 96% of people aged below 24. Van Deursen and Helsper (2015) revealed that many older adults who do not use the internet are not eager and interested in doing so. Other factors include technophobia, cognitive deficit, perceived lack of usefulness (Horrigan, 2010; Wu et al., 2015) and family influence (Friemel, 2016).

This digital divide may lead to double exclusion as the pandemic has led to limited physical social contact given the government-imposed total lockdown and subsequent movement restrictions and continuous social distancing. Several studies have shown that loneliness has increased within the older population as a result of the pandemic (Berg-Weger & Morley, 2020; Brooke & Jackson, 2020; Simard & Volicer, 2020; WHO, 2020; Wu, 2020) because older people tend to be excluded from in-person social contact especially in a traditional society like Nigeria where social contact is very important to older people (Ebimgbo et al., 2019), and they also belong to the group who often lack access to internet communication or decide against the use of new technologies (Gibson et al., 2020; Seifert, 2020) at a time when young people have turned to internet use to cope with the pandemic-induced social separation (Hamilton et al., 2020; Mukhtar, 2020; Vogels, 2020). In addition to communication with people, this lack of internet use may disenfranchise and deprive older people of useful online services and contents such as health information, digital social events, online shopping and social networking, healthcare delivery and services (Gibson et al., 2020; McDonough, 2016; Seifert, 2020); they may also lose the mental health benefit of internet use which was found to enhance psychological wellbeing among older users (Erb, 2014; Mukhtar, 2020).

Scholars like Nimrod (2020), Robinson et al. (2020), and Rorai and Perry (2020) have argued that the digital divide will pose new risks for vulnerable populations like older people during the pandemic as they may become more socially excluded, and face isolation and loneliness, while Banskota et al. (2020), Giwa et al. (2020), and Xie et al. (2020) posited that this is the time when going digital is crucial for the information, service and social inclusion needs of older people. Also, Henning-Smith (2020) argued that older people in rural communities may face more severe social implications of the COVID-19 pandemic, not only as a result of the health risk of the virus, but of not being able to meet their healthcare, social, and basic needs due to limited access to technology and internet connectivity. However, majority of the literature cited were commentaries and theoretical studies from scholars in the Global North. Thus, this study will be the first to empirically explore how older people in rural communities in Nigeria who might be digitally excluded have been coping with loneliness induced by the pandemic. This will help gerontological social workers understand the peculiar social contact needs of older people in rural Nigeria and provide needed support.

Materials and methods

We adopted a qualitative design for this study which afforded us the opportunity to deeply explore (Bryman, 2016) the experience of selected older adults in rural Nigeria with regards to the social effects of the pandemic-induced restrictions on them. We conducted this study inductively to allow themes and findings flow freely from the data and to resist the temptation of trying to force findings to fit into a preselected theoretical framework (Gobena & Hean, 2019).

Sample and recruitment

The study was centered on older adults (60 years and older) resident in rural Nigeria. Thus, the empirical material for the study was collected from 11 older adults in Ihe community, Awgu Local Government Area of Enugu State, Southeast Nigeria. Using purposive sampling technique, we selected older adults who were willing to discuss their experience with us in great detail (Bryman, 2016). Participants were chosen in such a way that different age groups (60s, 70s, 80s), genders, levels of education and occupations were represented. The choice of 11 participants was suitable in our small-scale qualitative study as it allowed for saturation and manageable data (Cresswell & Poth, 2018; Nelson, 2017), while the differences in certain demographic characteristics allowed for some diversity in participants' perspectives.

Recruitment for participation was relatively easy because the study was conducted in the indigenous community of one of the authors. He spoke to

Table 1. Demographic characteristics of participants.

Pseudonyms	Age	Gender	Level of education	Occupation	Living arrangement
Michael	80	M	No formal education	Retired	Children
Joy	71	F	No formal education	Retired	Alone
Jack	65	M	Primary education	Farmer	Spouse and children
Vivian	70	F	Primary education	Trader	Children
Jane	65	F	Undergraduate education	Retired	Alone
Cynthia	73	F	No formal education	Retired	Alone
Amanda	81	F	No formal education	Retired	Children
Peter	66	M	Primary education	Farmer	Spouse
Mary	76	F	No formal education	Retired	Children
Paul	72	M	Primary education	Farmer	Alone
Charles	69	M	Secondary education	Trader	Spouse and children

Source: *Data collected on digital and physical exclusion of older adults in Nigeria, 2020.*

as many older adults as he could about our project, giving them detailed information about the study and asking if they were willing to participate.

Table 1 shows that the 11 older adults who were chosen to participate in the study included 5 men and 6 women aged between 60 to 81 years. Four participants lived alone while seven lived with family (spouse and/or children). Six of the 11 older adults were retired, three were farmers and two were traders. The level of education shows that five participants did not have any formal education, four had primary education, two had secondary education and only one had undergraduate education. All 11 older adults participated of their own volition.

Data collection

Data for the study was collected using semi-structured in-depth interviews. We chose interviews because of their suitability for studies focused on exploring participants' experience and understanding of a given phenomenon (Bryman, 2016; Hammersley & Atkinson, 2007). The semi-structured nature of the interviews was a great fit for this study's inductive design, allowing the direction of the discussions go toward issues raised by participants during the interviews. The interviews were conducted in Igbo language and recorded electronically. Notes were taken during and after the interviews to complement the recordings.

The interviews were conducted during the first wave of the pandemic. Thus, anti-infection measures were put in place to protect the older adults, as they fall within the high-risk group vulnerable to the virus. Both during the recruitment phase and the interview itself, a distance of about 2 meters was kept between the interviewer/speaker and the older adults. Discussions were held in an open space, outside the homes of the older adults, and facemasks were worn by all parties, which caused some audibility issues because everyone had to speak louder than usual for clarity.

Data collection was conducted in line with ethical requirements for qualitative research: giving participants detailed information about the study and obtaining their consent before their participation, ensuring the interviews were conducted in a space, manner and language that guaranteed their safety, comfortability and full participation, and abiding by anti-infection guidelines during the data collection (Bryman, 2016; Pittaway et al., 2010). Ethical approval for the study was gotten from a certified Ethics Board in Nigeria.

Analysis

The recorded data was transcribed following a denaturalized transcription method since the study was focused on perspectives and meanings created and shared (Oliver et al., 2005) by older adults concerning social exclusionary effects of social distancing measures. Denaturalization allowed the focus of the transcription to be the content of the interviews i.e., what was said and not on linguistic features, accents, grammatical errors and verbal idiosyncrasies (Oliver et al., 2005). Although the interviews were conducted in Igbo language, using the parallel transcription framework by Nikander (2008), they were transcribed in English language, staying as close as possible to participants' original statements in Igbo. The transcribed versions were then compared with the recorded discussions by the researchers to ensure participants' original meanings and ideas were retained and to guarantee validity of data (Kalof et al., 2008).

Participants were pseudonymized after the transcription to ensure anonymity and confidentiality. For instance, the label 'Mary, F, 76' represent a seventy-six-year older female participant with the pseudonym 'Mary'. After the transcription, we employed thematic analytical method to analyze the data, and this involved using data to discover, interpret and report meaning patterns (Braun & Clarke, 2006). One of the researchers specialized in the use of Nvivo 12 software coded the data and shared the coding with the other researchers. We reflected on the interviewees' narratives by conducting multiple reads of both individual transcripts and the entire interview, comparing it with the Nvivo coding to identify emerging themes and also ensure validity, reliability and trustworthiness of the results. Inductive approach during the coding and analysis was adopted, having no preexisting code outline and immersing ourselves in the data through multiple readings of the transcripts until we saw emerging codes and patterns which were then organized in themes (Bryman, 2016). We wrote the findings using selected quotes from the interviews as supporting evidence.

Results

The pandemic has not only affected the social life of older people in urban areas but also of those in rural communities in Nigeria. Two major themes emerged from the findings of this study: the first theme illustrates how the pandemic-induced lockdown, restrictions and social distancing have deprived older people of social contact and led to loneliness, while the second theme shows how unlike younger people, many older people are largely unable to adopt the use of digital technology to cope with the pandemic, leading to double exclusion.

Pandemic-induced loneliness

Social contact with family, neighbors and friends is important for the emotional and psychological wellbeing of older people. However, anti-infection measures instituted against the COVID-19 pandemic such as social distancing, lockdown and movement restrictions are anti-social-contact by design. This has reduced contact between older people in rural areas and their children who normally visit them from the urban centers. Analysis shows that the two major factors that have contributed to limited social contact with family and friends were the lockdown and movement restrictions, and the economic fallout of the pandemic which has reduced their children's income.

During the lockdown, the government ordered everyone to stay in their homes *"people stayed away because of government instructions"* (Jack, M, 65), thus older adults' children who live away from them were not allowed to visit their parents. Lifting the lockdown started with movement for essential services and supplies, at this point people were allowed to go to the market for supplies within a specific period of time, 8am to 4pm in many states in Nigeria. People were still not allowed to travel, and state borders were closed. Consequently, many urban dwellers were not allowed to travel to rural communities. Therefore, older people's family members in the urban areas could still not visit them after the lockdown was lifted. Findings also revealed that the advice by the government and medical experts for maintenance of social distancing further limited social contact between older people and their neighbors and friends. This lack of social contact made many older people in the rural areas feel lonely during and after the lockdown with one participant even stating that the loneliness will adversely affect their health *"I don't see my children. It made me feel lonely and feeling lonely is a very big disease"* (Vivian, F, 70). Jane recounted:

> Is there anyone going to people's houses this period? Everyone stays indoor, I cook the little thing I see and I'm alone. The government insisted we stay at home to be safe, even when they said we should come out, they still said we should stay far from others. The

Igwe [Traditional Ruler] even brought some people who advised us to stay away from others (Jane, F, 65).

Findings also indicated that even after the lockdown and movement restrictions have been relaxed by the government, older people in rural communities continue to experience limited social contact from their family members. This is as a result of the economic fallout of the COVID-19 pandemic. It is customary for children to bring material goods to their parents in the rural areas when they come to visit. But the economic strain caused by the pandemic has made it difficult for people to buy material goods which they will take to their aging parents in the rural area, so they prefer to remain in the urban centers until their economic status increases. In extreme cases, some participants reported that their children cannot visit them because they cannot afford to pay the cost of transportation from urban to rural areas.

> Since this corona thing started my children have been complaining that there is no money. I asked my son when he will come and see me and he said 'father, will I come to see you empty handed?' He doesn't have money to buy the things he will bring for me. I was just telling him that I want to see him even if he doesn't give me anything, but he won't listen to me (Jack, M, 65).

> There is no money anywhere, even us in the village, we have noticed that things are now more expensive and there is still no money. Will I give my child money to come and see me? It should be the other way round, my child should be giving me money, but now he said he doesn't even have money for transportation from Onitsha (Cynthia, F, 73).

The ban on social gatherings such as churches, weddings and burial ceremonies also contribute in making older people in rural areas lonely. Older people in rural communities attend social events to socialize and interact with other people in the community. Sometimes, their children and other relatives return to the rural areas when there is an event like a wedding or burial, but the government's ban on social gathering put it to an end, thus making older people in rural communities stay alone in their homes.

> I can't even go to church to pray to God so that he will protect us from all these things. The whole world is paying for their sins. We don't even go to weddings and things like that again, our people don't come back anymore, we don't see people in the city anymore (Amanda, F, 81).

Digital exclusion

Older people do not use digital technology and internet as much as younger people do, and this is even worse for older people who reside in rural areas with limited electricity, internet connections and digital devices. All the participants in this study reported not having a smart phone *"I don't have it oh, but some people do show me things that happens in there"* (Vivian, F, 70).

Some of them stated that they would like to own a smart phone in order connect to their children and relatives through Facebook and WhatsApp, but they cannot afford to buy smart phones. Some stated that they barely have electricity and will not be able to power smartphones if they are able to get one. Jane, who is retired teacher, stated:

> I heard that I can even be seeing my children on the phone if I have that kind of phone, but I cannot afford to buy that kind of phone. If my children can buy it for me, it will be good oh. At least I will be seeing them whenever I want (Jane, F, 65).

While Peter insisted:

> In this village, we don't always have light [electricity]. How will I charge the phone if I have a phone? I can't start going to look for where to charge the phone like all these children. They should start giving us constant electricity first before you talk about us using phones (Peter, M, 66).

Findings also revealed that the digital divide is as a result of lack skills in using new digital technologies. Participants argued that even if they have access to digital technology and the internet, they lack the technical knowhow to take advantage of it. A female participant who is retired teacher indicated that if she has someone who will teach her how to use digital gadgets, she would love to surf the web, read news and watch videos online: *"I would have loved to be seeing things on phone too, both on WhatsApp, if they teach me"* (Jane, F, 65). Marry added:

> My son, I didn't even go to school, how will I start using things like that? I am too old to start learning such things. E ma na anaghi amu aka ekpe na nka [you know one doesn't learn to become ambidextrous at old age]. The only thing I know is that whenever I want to talk to my children, I carry this book and give to one of these children to call any of my children for me (Mary, F, 76).

Finally, some of the sampled participants did not report feeling left out because of the digital divide. Some participants totally rejected new digital technology, insisting that it is for children. Some of the sampled older adults argued that the use of digital devices and the internet is for young people because they didn't grow up with it *" . . . the children do make use of their phones but for me, I can't make use of it"* (Peter, M, 66). The older adults' generation grew up with radios so many of them tend to be only comfortable using radios: *"the one I have (laughs), I only have radio"* (Paul, M, 72). Listening to radios was adopted by many rural older people, especially older men; one of the participants stated that while he sees his daughter keeping herself busy by either making TikTok videos or watching TikTok video, he keeps himself busy by listening to his FM radio. The older women barely listened to radio, some of them said that farming, maintaining the house and doing house chores kept them busy during the lockdown. Many rural older women are housewives who stay at home, hence, maintaining the home has always been part of their everyday lives.

... it didn't make me feel bad because I didn't grow up with it and I don't know anything about it. Our age mates don't know anything about that ... I can't explain because they (younger people) spend all their time with their phones, I don't know what they're pressing on the phone and I can't tell them to stop using their phones. But for me, my radio is enough for me (Paul, M, 72).

My last child, the girl. She is always videoing herself or watching video with her phone and she will be laughing. One day I asked her why she is always videoing herself when she is doing anything. She will video herself dancing, singing, even eating, ha ha ha. She said it is titpop (interviewer: TikTok?), Yes. I don't know why you children do those things (Jack, M, 65).

Despite the recognized digital divide between older people in the rural communities in Nigeria and younger persons and the identified loneliness caused by the pandemic. Some older people in rural Nigeria do not perceive themselves as digitally excluded, they view the use of new digital technology as a child's plaything: *"no I can't feel bad about that I'm not a child"* (Paul, M, 72). The older adults did not acknowledge that bridging the digital divide will make them less lonely in the face of the pandemic: *"no, I don't think it will help"* (Paul, M, 72). Therefore, while there is need to address the pandemic-induced loneliness among older people in rural community, this may not be achieved through digital interventions.

Discussion

Our study explored the views of 11 older adults in rural Nigeria on the social exclusion resulting from restrictions introduced to control the spread of the COVID-19; contributing to the growing body of literature on older adults and standing as the first empirical effort to explore the exclusionary effects of the pandemic on older adults in rural Nigeria. Our analysis of in-depth interviews conducted with the older adults revealed that many suffer from pandemic-induced loneliness (Berg-Weger & Morley, 2020; Brooke & Jackson, 2020; Simard & Volicer, 2020; WHO, 2020; Wu, 2020) and digital exclusion (Seifert, 2020). Many of the older adults face double exclusion and double loneliness, but some manage to stay connected using other media.

Movement and social proximity restrictions introduced in many countries have had extreme exclusionary effects on those belonging to high-risk groups. Because of their advanced age and vulnerability to serious complications from COVID-19, older adults have had to live under stricter social distancing measures compared to the rest of the population (Simard & Volicer, 2020; Wu, 2020), which implies being largely excluded from the society as they know it. Older adults who participated in this study reported being physically excluded from contacts with their children, families and social networks, making it difficult for them to access the needed social, emotional and economic support.

While many people around the world, especially younger people, are able to make up for the pandemic-induced physical social exclusion using digital technologies and social media (Hamilton et al., 2020; Mukhtar, 2020; Vogels, 2020), many older adults in rural areas are unable to, because of digital illiteracy (Blažič & Blažič, 2020), restricted access to these technologies (Formosa, 2013; Rorai & Perry, 2020), poor electricity and internet connectivity (Roberts, 2010) and plain disinterest in new technologies (Gibson et al., 2020; Van Deursen & Helsper, 2015). Older adults from our study are unable to use Zoom and video calls to stay connected to loved ones they have been restricted from seeing and talking to, or to use TikTok, Instagram and Facebook as media to connect to a larger network and be reminded that "we are all in this together". In facing restricted physical and digital contact with their social networks, many of these older adults suffer double social exclusion.

The limited physical social contact with families and social networks has led to increased loneliness within the older population (Berg-Weger & Morley, 2020; Brooke & Jackson, 2020; Simard & Volicer, 2020; WHO, 2020; Wu, 2020). This loneliness is especially extreme in contexts like Nigeria where social contact is vital to the wellbeing of older adults (Ebimgbo et al., 2019). The older adults who participated in this study reported feeling extremely lonely because people stay away from them (although to protect them), they are unable to see their children and loved ones, and they cannot attend social events and religious fellowships which serve as a major source of strength and community for them.

Although many older adults reported being unable to use digital technologies and connections to counter the physical exclusion and resulting loneliness brought on by the pandemic (Hamilton et al., 2020; Mukhtar, 2020; Vogels, 2020), some were indifferent about this. For them, it was a case of not missing what one never had. Older adults who lack interest in digital technologies (Rorai & Perry, 2020; Van Deursen & Helsper, 2015) or who possibly have not considered the ways these technologies can make up for physical social exclusion, neither feel digitally excluded nor face loneliness as a result of this. Some participants in this study reduce loneliness and stay connected to the world around them by listening to their FM radios while some older women use farm work and house chores to keep busy and fight loneliness. This shows that while it may be useful to bridge the digital divide existing between older people and younger people to control the risks of social exclusion and facilitate older people's access to information, social support and services available online (Banskota et al., 2020; Giwa et al., 2020; Henning-Smith, 2020; Nimrod, 2020; Robinson et al., 2020; Xie et al., 2020), there is a great potential in considering other resources, activities, ways of being and systems older adults in rural areas use to counter or reduce the social effects of the pandemic on them.

Limitations

The current pandemic posed limitations for this study as the researchers had to take extra caution to ensure the participants of this study were not put at the risk of getting infected. This contributed to the limited number of participants for this study (n = 11). However, this is a qualitative study which was not designed for generalization but to get detailed and in-depth views about the subject matter, thus, we recommend interpretation of findings with caution. We recognize that statistical significance is a good indicator of the potential validity of findings, therefore, it is important to note our findings may not be generalizable to the larger population. To improve validity and reliability of our research findings, we used a standardized methodology, conducted the study in a familiar context, did not incentivize participants, had no predetermined research findings, did not focus on generalization but on rich descriptions of the research context and participants to allow for comparisons with other contexts in which transfer may be contemplated (Bailey, 2007; Gobena & Hean, 2019)

Recommendations

Although, our study shows that some older people do not perceive digital exclusion as contributing to their social isolation and loneliness, all the participants in the study identified that the pandemic has increased social isolation and loneliness. Therefore, there is need to keep older people encouraged and motivated without the use of digital technology. The use of mainstream media, such as radio and television, was identified to help older people cope with the pandemic, thus those who work with them should include contents focused on older people and encourage them to express themselves through live calls. Older people should also be encouraged to participate in live broadcasts of religious fellowships as many religious institutions now broadcast their sermons on radio and television stations in Nigeria.

Caregivers, family members and gerontological social workers should maintain regular phone contact with homebound older people to provide friendship while family members of literate older people can send letters and cards to their parents. The Nigerian government should set up a mental health hotline which will not only receive calls but also add outgoing calls so that mental health professionals can reach out to older people in rural communities and screen for depressive and anxiety symptoms.

Finally, older people should be encouraged to engage in day-to-day activities that will benefit their spiritual, mental and physical wellbeing on their own, especially those at the risk of delirium. They can engage in light physical activities at home, and their children can help them create an engaging daily schedule to keep them active. Older people can also engage in outdoor activities while keeping strictly to social distancing measures. Exposure to sunlight and the feel of the outdoors can be beneficial for their wellbeing.

ORCID

Prince Chiagozie Ekoh ⓘ http://orcid.org/0000-0002-1787-536X
Elizabeth Onyedikachi George ⓘ http://orcid.org/0000-0001-5678-4113
Chigozie Donatus Ezulike ⓘ http://orcid.org/0000-0002-7883-5679

References

Age UK. (2018). *Policy position paper: Digital inclusion.* https://www.ageuk.org.uk/globalassets/age-uk/documents/policy-positions/active-communities/ppp_digital-_inclusion_uk.pdf

Anderson, M., Perrin, A., Jiang, J., & Kumar, M. (2019). *10% of Americans don't use the internet. Who are they?* Pew Research Center. https://www.pewresearch.org/fact-tank/2019/04/22/some-americans-dont-use-the-internet-who-are-they/

Bailey, C. A. (2007). *A guide to qualitative field research* (2nd ed.). Pine Forge Press. https://doi.org/10.4135/9781412983204

Banskota, S., Healy, M., & Goldberg, E. M. (2020). 15 Smartphone apps for older adults to use while in isolation during the COVID-19 pandemic. *Western Journal of Emergency Medicine, 21*(3), 514–525. https://doi.org/10.5811/westjem.2020.4.47372

Berg-Weger, M., & Morley, J. E. (2020). Loneliness and social isolation in older adults during the Covid-19 pandemic: Implications for gerontological social work. *The Journal of Nutrition, Health & Aging, 24*(5), 456–458. https://doi.org/https://doi.org/https://doi.org/10.1007/s12603-020-1366-8

Blažič, B. J., & Blažič, A. J. (2020). Overcoming the digital divide with a modern approach to learning digital skills for the elderly adults. *Education and Information Technologies, 25*(1), 259–279. https://doi.org/10.1007/s10639-019-09961-9

Braun, V., & Clarke, V. (2006). Using thematic analysis in psychology. *Qualitative Research in Psychology, 3*(2), 77–101. https://doi.org/10.1191/1478088706qp063oa

Brooke, J., & Jackson, D. (2020). Older people and COVID-19: Isolation, risk and ageism. *Journal of Clinical Nursing, 29*(13–14), 2044–2046. https://doi.org/10.1111/jocn.15274

Bryman, A. (2016). *Social research methods* (5th ed.). Oxford University Press.

Centre for Ageing Better. (2018). *The digital age: New approaches to support people in later life get online.* https://www.ageing-better.org.uk/sites/default/files/2018-05/The-digital-age.pdf

Cresswell, J. W., & Poth, C. N. (2018). *Qualitative inquiry and research design: Choosing among five approaches* (4th ed.). SAGE Publications.

Ebimgbo, S. O., Obi-Keguna, C. N., Chukwu, N. E., Onalu, C. E., Abonyi, S. E., & Okoye, U. O. (2019). Culture-bases social support to older adults in Nnewi, South-East Nigeria. *African Population Studies, 33*(2), 4891–4900. https://doi.org/10.11564/33-2-1402

Erb, R. (2014). *Teaching seniors to use Internet cuts depression risk.* Detroit Free Press.

Formosa, M. (2013). Digital exclusion in later life: A Maltese case study. *Humanities and Social Sciences, 1*(1), 21–27. https://doi.org/10.11648/j.hss.20130101.14

Friemel, T. N. (2016). The digital divide has grown old: Determinants of a digital divide among seniors. *New Media & Society, 18*(2), 313–331. https://doi.org/10.1177/1461444814538648

Gibson, A., Bardach, S. H., & Pope, D. N. (2020). COVID-19 and the digital divide: Will social workers help bridge the gap? *Journal of Gerontological Social Work*, *63*(6–7), 671–673. https://doi.org/10.1080/01634372.2020.1772438

Giwa, S., Mullings, D. V., & Karki, K. (2020). Virtual social work care with older black adults: A culturally relevant technology-based intervention to reduce social isolation and loneliness in a time of pandemic. *Journal of Gerontological Social Work*, *63*(6–7), 679–681. https://doi.org/10.1080/01634372.2020.1800885

Gobena, E. B., & Hean, S. C. (2019). The experience of incarcerated mothers living in a correctional institution with their children in Ethiopia. *Journal of Comparative Social Work*, *14*(2), 30–54. https://doi.org/10.31265/jcsw.v14.i2.247

Hamilton, J. L., Nesi, J., & Choukas-Bradley, S. (2020). *Teens and social media during the COVID-19 pandemic: Staying socially connected while physically distant*. PsyArXiv Preprints. https://doi.org/10.31234/osf.io/5stx4

Hammersley, M., & Atkinson, P. (2007). *Ethnography: Principles in practice* (3rd ed.). Routledge Taylor and Francis Group.

Henning-Smith, C. (2020). The unique impact of COVID-19 on older adults in rural areas. *Journal of Aging & Social Policy*, *32*(4–5), 396–402. https://doi.org/10.1080/08959420.2020.1770036

Horrigan, J. B. (2010). *Broadband adoption & use in America: Results from an FCC survey*. Federal Communications Commission.

Hunsaker, A., & Hargittai, E. (2018). A review of internet use among older adults. *New Media & Society*, *20*(10), 3937–3954. https://doi.org/10.1177/1461444818787348

Kalof, L., Dan, A., & Dietz, T. (2008). *Essential of social research*. Open University Press.

McDonough, C. C. (2016). The effect of ageism on the digital divide among older adults. *Journal of Gerontology & Geriatric Medicine*, *2*(1), 008. https://doi.org/10.24966/GGM-8662/100008

Mukhtar, S. (2020). Psychosocial impact of COVID-19 on older adults: A cultural geriatric mental health-care perspective. *Journal of Gerontological Social Work*, *63*(6–7), 665–667. https://doi.org/10.1080/01634372.2020.1779159

Nelson, J. (2017). Using conceptual depth criteria: Addressing the challenge of reaching saturation in qualitative research. *Quality Research*, *17*(5), 554–570. https://doi.org/10.1177%2F1468794116679873

Nikander, P. (2008). Working with transcripts and translated data. *Qualitative Research in Psychology*, *5*(3), 225–231. https://doi.org/10.1080/14780880802314346

Nimrod, G. (2020). Changes in internet use when coping with stress: Older adults during the COVID-19 pandemic. *The American Journal of Geriatric Psychiatry*, *28*(10), 1020–1024. https://doi.org/10.1016/j.jagp.2020.07.010

Office for National Statistics. (2018). *Dataset: Internet users*. https://www.ons.gov.uk/file?uri=%2fbusinessindustryandtrade%2fitandinternetindustry%2fdatasets%2finternetusers%2fcurrent/finaltables2019.xlsx

Oliver, D. G., Serovich, J. M., & Mason, T. L. (2005). Constraints and opportunities with interview transcription: Towards reflection in qualitative research. *Social Forces*, *84*(2), 1273–1289. https://doi.org/10.1353/sof.2006.0023

Pittaway, E., Bartolomei, L., & Hugman, R. (2010). Stop stealing our stories: The ethics of research with vulnerable groups. *Journal of Human Rights Practice*, *2*(2), 229–251. https://doi.org/10.1093/jhuman/huq004

Roberts, S. (2010). *The fictions, facts and future of older people and technology*. International Longevity Centre.

Robinson, L., Schulz, J., Khilnani, A., Ono, H., Cotten, S. R., McClain, N., Levine, L., Chen, W., Huang, G., Casilli, A. A., Tubaro, P., Dodel, M., Quan-Haase, A., Ruiu, M. L., Ragnedda, M.,

Aikat, D., & Tolentino, N. (2020). Digital inequalities in time of pandemic: COVID-19 exposure risk profiles and new forms of vulnerability. *First Monday*, *25*(7), 1-34. https://doi.org/10.5210/fm.v25i7.10845

Rorai, V., & Perry, T. E. (2020). An Innovative telephone outreach program to seniors in Detroit, a city facing dire consequences of COVID-19. *Journal of Gerontological Social Work*, *63*(6–7), 713–716. https://doi.org/10.1080/01634372.2020.1793254

Seifert, A. (2020). The digital exclusion of older adults during the COVID-19 pandemic. *Journal of Gerontological Social Work*, *63*(6–7), 674–676. https://doi.org/10.1080/01634372.2020.1764687

Simard, J., & Volicer, L. (2020). Loneliness and isolation in long-term care and the Covid-19 pandemic. *Journal of the American Medical Directors Association*, *21*(7), 966–967. https://doi.org/10.1016/j.jamda.2020.05.006

van Bronswijk, J. E., Fozard, J. L., Kearns, W. D., Davison, G. C., & Tuan, P. C. (2008). Implementing gerontechnology. *Gerontechnology*, *7*(3), 325–327. https://doi.org/10.4017/gt.2008.07.03.007.00

Van Deursen, A., & Helsper, E. (2015). A nuanced understanding of Internet use and non-use amongst older adults. *European Journal of Communication*, *30*(2), 171–187. https://doi.org/10.1177/0267323115578059

Vogels, E. A. (2020). *From virtual parties to ordering food, how Americans are using the internet during COVID19*. Pew Research Center. https://www.pewresearch.org/fact-tank/2020/04/30/from-virtual-parties-to-ordering-food-how-americans-are-using-the-internet-during-covid-19/

WHO. (2020). *Mental health and psychosocial considerations during the COVID-19 outbreak*. https://www.who.int/docs/default-source/coronaviruse/mental-health-considerations.pdf?sfvrsn=6d3578af_2

Wu, B. (2020). Social isolation and loneliness among older adults in the context of COVID-19: A global challenge. *Global Health Research and Policy*, *5*(1), 27. https://doi.org/10.1186/s41256-020-00154-3

Wu, Y. H., Damnée, S., Kerhervé, H., Ware, C., & Rigaud, A. S. (2015). Bridging the digital divide in older adults: A study from an initiative to inform older adults about new technologies. *Clinical Interventions in Aging*, *2015*(10), 193–200. https://doi.org/10.2147/CIA.S72399

Xie, B., Charness, N., Fingerman, K., Kaye, J., Kim, M. T., & Khurshid, A. (2020). When going digital becomes a necessity: Ensuring older adults' needs for information, services, and social inclusion during COVID-19. *Journal of Aging & Social Policy*, *32*(4–5), 460–470. https://doi.org/10.1080/08959420.2020.1771237

Yang, J., & Du, P. (2020). Gender, capital endowment and digital exclusion of older people in China. *Ageing and Society*, 1–25. https://doi.org/10.1017/S0144686X20000434

Digital Inclusion of Older Adults during COVID-19: Lessons from a Case Study of Older Adults Technology Services (OATS)

Joyce Weil ⓘ, Thomas Kamber, Alexander Glazebrook, Marisa Giorgi and Kimberly Ziegler

ABSTRACT

Older adults' relationship to information and communications technology (ICT) is often discussed in terms of the digital divide or technology gap. Older persons, those 65 years of age and older, are seen as excluded or marginally represented in the digital sphere, even though data show their use of technology is increasing. Challenges in technology adoption and models for improving digital inclusion are both well-known, but the COVID pandemic and its general shift to digital life have created a critical need to increase digital inclusion of older persons. A case study of Older Adults Technology Services (OATS) and the organization's migration from in-person to virtual programming is used as an example of reframing the way the relationship of older adults to technology is seen in the field and in practice. Policy and programming implications of this new view of technology are discussed in the conclusion.

Introduction

Older adults' information and communications technology (ICT) use is often discussed in terms of the digital divide, highlighting those excluded from the digital sphere. The digital divide concept was developed to illustrate the potential impact of technology access by creating two distinct groups: those with it, "the haves," and those without, "the have nots" (National Telecommunication and Information Administration, 1994). Early gerotechnologists (also called gerontechnologists) suggested that the digital divide is not a static state, and since the 1980s, the field of gerontechnology has worked to increase technology access and adoption for older adults (Kwon, 2017). Charness and Holley (2004) suggested, at that time, "the leading edge of the baby boom generation is just now moving into their late 50s. Today's seniors are generally nonusers of new media. Tomorrow's seniors are likely to be avid users" (p. 428).

While internet access and use may differ by older age cohorts (those 65–74, 75–84, and 85 years of age) and other sociodemographic factors, rates for those 65 years of age and older are increasing over time (Seifert et al., 2020). According to a Pew Research Institute Report, in 2019, 73% of those over 65 years of age use the internet. About 59% of older adults have broadband services at home with only 12% relying on a smartphone alone to access the internet at home without broadband. As a comparison, using the youngest age group in the Pew Report, 100% of those 18–29 years of age use the internet. About 77% of this group have broadband services at home with 22% relying on a smartphone alone to access the internet at home without broadband (Pew Research Center, 2019). While older adults who lack access to technology and/ or have lower levels of adoption are often referred to as being in the "digital divide," or even as part of the "grey digital divide" (intended to highlight their older age as a factor), the impact of lack of access must be understood as more nuanced than the inability to access broadband; access to technology offers social inclusion, lifelong learning opportunities, and connection to financial and many other resources (Glazebrook, 2020).

Older adults can gain a sense of empowerment when they successfully migrate these in-person experiences to the digital sphere (Estes, 2019; Lind et al., 2020). The COVID-19 pandemic and its increased social isolation among older adults has prompted a need to examine and reframe aspects of the "divide" to increase digital literacy and inclusion of older adults living in the community (Glazebrook, 2020).

Reframing older adults' relationship to technology

Understanding ways to increase digital inclusion is even more vital as the COVID pandemic has brought a general shift and migration to digital life. There is a need to encourage more robust participation in ICT and increased access to broadband at home. Researchers have found that older adults sheltering in place in their homes during COVID-19 may experience isolation from their social networks of family and friends (Armitage & Nellums, 2020). With the shift to completing daily tasks digitally, older adults reported feeling unable to meet their daily needs. Difficulty meeting these Instrumental Activities of Daily Living (IADLs, such as home and financial management and getting daily necessities) in a virtual mode left older adults stating they feel like a "burden" to others – which led to high levels of distress (Losada-Baltar et al., 2020). At various times throughout the pandemic of COVID-19, in-person services and community-based resources were often closed, leaving many older adults seeking essentials like food, medication, and healthcare in new ways, including online (Xie et al., 2020). Researchers suggest that more long-term effects of COVID-19 over an older adult's life course could include changes in: feelings of personal control, relating to family and friends, patterns of work, and seeking education and training (Settersten et al., 2020; Zubatsky et al., 2020). Older adults may feel less agency or control overall, see family and friends less often or virtually, be more likely to work virtually or lose face-to-face work, and seek additional life-long education and training in online settings (Chatterjee & Yatnatti, 2020). Older adults' inclusion in the digital sphere offers access to a comprehensive set of activities, from day-to-day online shopping and banking to use of social media and video chat to maintain social connections.

Empirical research has also explored barriers and gateways that influence older adults' use of technology. Barriers are based on age-related changes and socio-cultural factors. Studies summarize those physical-change-based barriers as: age-related changes in vision, hearing, dexterity, etc. (Kwon, 2017; Spears & Zheng, 2020). ICT are often not designed for older users in terms of font, color-choices, and layout (Weil, 2017). Socio-cultural factors that act as barriers include older adults' beliefs of limited perceived benefits of ICT, fear of stigma when learning, lack of age-inclusive training, personality and cognitive traits, and financial cost (Blaschke et al., 2009; Davidson et al., 2012; Hou et al., 2017; Kamber, 2017; Kamin et al., 2017; Yusif et al., 2016). Recent research has found that prior computer use and better financial status predict older adults' feelings of self-efficacy in computer and internet use (Spears & Zheng, 2020).

At the same time, models have been created to address defined barriers and increase technology adoption. For example, the Unified Theory of Acceptance and Use of Technology (UTAUT) includes comprehensive factors that influence intention to use technology (Venkatesh et al., 2003). This model shows the relationship between background characteristics and behavioral intention that leads to the final outcome of behavioral use. Characteristics – such as a person's belief that technology will help them do tasks, their perceived ease of learning, believing others feel learning technology is important, and that there will be real support in the learning process – affect behavioral intention to learn technology leading to positive technology-use behavior.

Research about how older adults learn successfully in online environments and virtual courses is still emerging. In a study of participants of multiple age groups taking Massive Open Online Courses (MOOCs), Xiong and Zuo (2019) found older adults may prefer a slower pace than different age groups and need more practice. In a virtual setting, as compared to an in-person one, older adults are more likely to have an intrinsic motivation for participation to learn rather than learning to meet an external goal. Xiong and Zuo (2019) found six key motivations for older adults who participate in online learning, including solving problems, acquiring knowledge, improving cognition, seeking fun, benefiting others, and keeping social contact. These motivations differed by age group and gender, but the "improving cognition" and "seeking fun" reasons were found to be unique to older learners. The authors also made several key recommendations that apply to an online learning environment for older adults: virtual programming should have an indication of progress throughout the course with reminders, a Q&A section or forum, recommendations at the end of the course for other courses that might interest the older-adult learner, quizzes/games to add interest, easy ways for the older adult to share course materials, and online discussion forums. In an online environment, older adults need real-life examples and context/explanation to know not only what they are learning, but why they need to know it (Xiong & Zuo, 2019).

The case study of Older Adult Technology Services (OATS), a nonprofit organization with a philosophy of using technology as a vehicle to empower older adults (Kamber, 2017), will be used to show the process of successful migration of older adults from in-person to virtual programming. It includes a discussion of the organization's in-person methodology, teaching practices, and course delivery, as well as how these were adapted to bring existing programming online to suit diverse groups of virtual learners (those already in the digital sphere and those new to virtual learning) and expand the curricular focus during COVID-19 to include a new set of needs and interests. Additionally, work by OATS in several collaborative virtual educational campaigns (e.g., the Association for the Advancement of Retired Persons, AARP, the New York Departments for the Aging and Housing Authority, DFTA, and NYCHA) is used to show the benefits and outcome of virtual learning for older adults. Findings from this digital migration will be used to reframe the way older adults are placed in the digital divide.

Case study

Pre-COVID-19, in-person, technology-based instruction

OATS sees technology as a vehicle for empowerment and an entry point for older adults seeking change in their lives and a new way to achieve their potential (Kamber, 2017; Kamin et al., 2017), measuring transformation in five impact areas: social engagement, health and wellness, financial security, civic participation, and creative expression. Integral to the OATS approach is its model of change, used in teaching ICT-based classes to older adults. As it defines itself, the organization is not about technology, *per se*; its model treats technology as an entry point for conversations and collaborations with older adults seeking change in their lives. Older adults who commit to personal change often seek new skills to achieve their goals. As part of this transformative experience, OATS creates an environment where older adults can achieve their potential or learn new skills.

From 2004 until March 15, 2020, OATS offered in-person technology classes to nearly 40,000 adults 60 and over, with a Net Promoter Score (NPS) – a measure of satisfaction and how likely someone is to recommend what they have experienced to another – of 81 (out of a possible score of 100) (Glazebrook & Sakow, 2020). The curriculum was guided by research-based principles to create course structure, format, and delivery. In-person courses were based on three methodologies: The OATS approach to curriculum design for Senior Planet programs, teaching methodology for Senior Planet programs, and training methodology for Senior Planet programs (Giorgi & Ziegler, 2019a, 2019b; Ziegler & Giorgi, 2019). "Senior Planet" refers to the website SeniorPlanet.org created in 2008. It began as an online content site for older adults, one that presents original feature stories, curated posts, and opportunities for commentaries related to interests of older adults and now also hosts virtual programming (Kamber, 2017; Kamin et al., 2017). During the pandemic, the site became the place to locate and access all virtual OATS content.

The guiding principle of the curriculum was based upon the methodological approach that learning is participant-based and inclusive with ample opportunity for hands-on application so participants can explore a topic in greater depth – through modeling and discussion. Course offerings included stand-alone lectures, workshops, and five- or ten-week classes. Courses were taught in a structured lesson format and time interval to groups of 10–15 older adults and included a written course book and paid trainer. Some of these classes were held at OATS centers or 24 OATS-created computer labs (via city and grant funding) within a network of more than 70 community-based organizations (e.g., community centers, senior centers).

OATS also developed Senior Planet U (SPU), an online learning platform, that remains active. SPU: "hosts a variety of online educational materials complementing in-person classes. This platform allows for a blended learning experience with multimedia content, promotes self-paced learning, and offers a flexible approach to when and where the learning takes place. Resources include articles, videos, interviews, and tutorials that correspond to the content in course books. Members retain access to SPU after the conclusion of a course" (OATS, 2020; Senior Planet Digital). Since 2004, outcome surveys were completed at the end of each course to measure impact of technology training with older adults. In 2013, the outcome survey was re-designed and psychometrically tested by a university-based researcher to capture data across the organization's five impact areas: health and wellness, civic engagement, creative expression, financial security, and social connectivity. To provide an overview of trends in these data, 20,000 responses over time show reductions in feelings of loneliness, increase in wellbeing, enhanced creativity, and better financial acuity. Additional survey details are available upon request (Glazebrook, 2020; OATS, 2021).

COVID-19 and the move to virtual programing

With NYC as one of the centers of the pandemic, by mid-March 2020 in-person operations at the Senior Planet Exploration Center were halted, as was in-person instruction in all OATS geographies. By early April, OATS had converted 20 lectures for delivery through SeniorPlanet.org and developed a virtual-programming framework. During this period, OATS staff began making phone calls to Senior Planet members across the United States to see how they were doing as the sheltering-in-place orders were enacted. In these months of the pandemic (mid-March through early-June), over 5,000 phone calls were made and 2,491 surveys collected. Telephone survey data collected during the calls gathered information about social engagement, general wellness, internet/broadband access, interest in connecting with other older adults, and virtual programming preferences. Survey data revealed that among Senior Planet participants: 16% had no internet access in their home, 37% desired help to get access set up, 77% were interested in online programming, and 34% were interested in pairing with other older adults to check in on one another (Glazebrook & Sakow, 2020).

Influenced by online learning pedagogy for older adults and prior experience with online learning through Senior Planet "Explore Tech" lectures (topical sessions on a variety of subjects), OATS sought to replicate the in-person experience as much as possible while being cognizant of the need to add interactive opportunities for participants so they could engage with the online sessions. Trainers, who previously taught in in-person classrooms, were also making the shift to teaching via Zoom – a format selected after other video learning platforms were considered. Piloting determined more time would be needed to give clear instructions to participants and for both trainers and participants to learn common features of the platform and technology used in the virtual classroom.

The OATS curriculum team designed and piloted materials using best virtual pedagogy practices for older adults – for example, adding additional discussion questions to each virtual class's structured slide presentation decks to build in more opportunities for participants' interaction. Or, increasing the length of time of a class to allow for a varied pace of learning in this new virtual classroom setting. Based on its virtual-inclusive teaching methodology, OATS developed materials that bridged the gap. In mid-March, the initial OATS lectures were converted for virtual delivery via Zoom to address older adults' need to access resources while sheltering in place. Some early topics included: food delivery apps, online grocery shopping, shopping on Amazon, online health resources, telehealth, online prescription-drug resources, and mindfulness apps. Other interactive presentations covered such topics as: peer-to-peer payments, protecting your personal information online, and online banking. Additionally, OATS created virtual series about how to use social media as a way to decrease social-isolation experiences during COVID-19. These materials – about messaging apps, video chat, and social media platforms (Facebook, Instagram, Twitter) – offer ways to build social connections safely while distancing.

As the pandemic continued, OATS has expanded its virtual programming to support all five of its impact areas (social engagement, health and wellness, financial security, civic participation, and creative expression). The content has also grown to include more social activities, tech-talks (pairing an older adult with a trainer knowledgeable about a specific technical topic for discussion and demonstration), and local special events. Table 1 includes the way key components of in-person courses and activities were transformed virtually. As of mid-August, more than 60 lectures and workshops have been converted from in-person Senior Planet content into virtual program offerings. Lectures run 60–75 minutes, depending upon their topic, and attendance ranges from 25–75 participants. Workshops, due to their "hands on" and more experiential nature, are intentionally designed to run longer and often have a range of 10–15 participants. OATS hotlines provide wraparound support before and after virtual program participation, allowing first-time technology users to build skills before participation. The hotline offers additional time for older adults with varying levels of digital literacy to work one-to-one with a trainer and practice. Open-lab sessions were added where participants could drop in the Zoom room and work on any skills they wanted to with a trainer.

Since the transition to virtual programming on March 16 until August 2020, OATS has taught more than 54,000 older adults online, with steady increase. Summary data for programs where an after-course survey was given offer an example of outcomes of the transition to virtual programming. As of mid-August 2020, 4,587 (of the approximately 14,800 possible) participants completed the post-course evaluation survey. The response rate was about 31%. The survey was administered via a Qualtrics link provided by trainers at the end of a session and available on the organization's website. A quick 5–10-minute, 13-question Qualtrics-based survey asked participants: if they participated in Senior Planet in person or virtual programming before, how they learned about Senior Planet, to give an overall rating of the class, to answer

Table 1. Converting in-person programming to virtual.

In-Person	Virtual

Stand-alone lectures and workshops
    5–10 week in-person courses
    (All impact areas)
	Lecture & Workshops
	    (individual, series)
	    (All impact areas)

Meeting with members in person at our sites	Social events: book club, crafting, member-led panels
Exercise classes on location	Zoom-based health and wellness

Technical help with a volunteer	Technical hotline
	    Video tutorials
	    COVID-19 resources on website
	    Zoom instructions

Likert questions about the impact of the class on their ability to connect with people, to list the devices they owned and ways they connected to the internet, and to offer suggestions about the class they attended. Of those who responded: 86% felt more connected to the world around them, and 78% were more confident connecting with friends and family online. Additionally, 82% felt better equipped to find resources online, and 80% felt less alone. The Net Promoter Score (NPS) is 94 (of a possible score of 100) across all virtual programs.

Collaborative virtual campaigns

In addition to its own virtual programming, OATS worked on virtual campaigns with several organizations. (The collaboration with AARP is used here as an example; see Table 2 for others.) In May 2020, AARP sought out OATS to design and deliver curricular materials for two topics: an introduction to Zoom and an overview of the benefits of having a my Social Security Account (mySSA.gov) during COVID-19. Two teams, one from each organization, met virtually and discussed ideas for each Zoom webinar. The curriculum team designed the materials and then worked to create a syllabus for a highly experienced trainer. AARP created scripts for videos featuring the trainer who also led five live Zoom webinars using the newly created curricular materials. Three sessions of "All Things Zoom" and two sessions of "Take Control of your Social Security Benefits" were offered from May-June 2020. All told, the collaboration with AARP served 20,344 older adults across the five sessions.

After each session, participants were sent a survey link. The survey had a response rate of 44% (n = 8,970). In terms of demographics, on average, attendees were 66.91 years of age (SD = 6.92), White (64%), and female (62%). Overall, 92% of respondents said they were either satisfied (57%) or very

Table 2. Virtual collaboration.

Organization	Timeline	Status/Outcome
Association for the Advancement of Retired Persons, AARP	May – June 2020	23,000+ participants learned to use Zoom and my Social Security Account (my SSA) Online
New York City Housing Authority, NYCHA, and Department for the Aging, DFTA	May 2020 – ongoing	Creation of tech call center by OATS to support education accompanying DFTA's free distribution of tablets. Ongoing rounds of 5-week educational series about how to use tablets via Zoom. 33,000+ calls to 10,000 older adults living alone
Zelle	May – July	Offered nonprofit expertise to collaborate with Zelle corporation to create and deliver online lectures and workshops about financial digital literacy via Zoom
Humana	June 2020 – ongoing	National connectivity initiative with a goal to connect 1 million older adults
Foster Grandparent Program and Grandparent Resource Center	August 1- ongoing	Make the tech hotline of OATS available for older adults volunteering to virtually mentor and connect with children and teenagers

satisfied (35%) with their experience of the virtual event. 94% said they were either likely (25%) or very likely (69%) to attend another virtual event hosted by AARP and Senior Planet.

When asked about which types of devices attendees own, the top three were: a working computer or laptop (38%), a smartphone (30%), and a tablet (17%). Fewer than 1% of those responding said "I do not have a device" which implies they are borrowing one to attend virtual programming. The top three ways that respondents connected to the internet were: through a cable internet connection in their home (60%), using the built-in LTE data plan on their smartphone (15%), or through a fiber-optic connection in their home (11%). Fewer than 1% said they do not connect to the internet. Referring back to general patterns of older adults and connectivity, AARP event attendees' access to the internet from home generally reflected the same trends seen in the Pew 2019 data. Overall, 61% of attendees have internet connection/broadband access at home like the 59% in Pew's survey. About 15% of the AARP webinar attendees rely on a smartphone alone to access the internet like the 12% in the Pew survey.

Practical lessons learned from the experience of OATS

The case study of OATS can lead to several recommendations at two levels, practice and policy, about improving digital inclusion rather than focusing on the digital divide. Lessons learned from the organization's reflections about its experience can help other organizations. These practice guidelines are discussed here, and policy recommendations are noted in the concluding section. This case study shows key aspects of transitioning older adults to the digital sphere. It requires training and sessions designed with the older learner in mind, iterative-based techniques based on evaluation and feedback by the older adults, and well-trained trainers who are knowledgeable about working with older adults so this experience can carry over to virtual learning. For other organizations in the process of migrating in-person programming for older adults to a virtual setting, adopting these practices can improve technology use. Namely, curriculum and modes of program delivery have to be redesigned for a variety of learners, and best practices need to be implemented to address the learning needs of each group. For example, it is helpful to create additional materials (such as handouts or videos) for those new to video chat platforms (such as Zoom) or offer a tech hotline phone number so older adults can talk with technology trainers about specific questions as they arise.

In terms of staffing, trainers or those presenting sessions online may find the virtual room harder to read than an in-person class. Having more presenters or co-presenters, in a team-based teaching approach, aids in assessing group dynamics and teaching learners at differing levels of digital literacy. While the main presenter can deliver the information, additional presenters can field chatted questions and provide further instruction to participants in smaller breakout-room settings. The additional presenter can scan the virtual room and give ongoing feedback to the main presenter about any topics that are unclear and require more explanation.

At an organizational level, responsiveness to older adults' interests and feedback is key. The use of surveys or other assessment instruments allows organizations to capture and evaluate participants' data. Ongoing multiple data points ensure that programming is dynamic and iterative. These assessments also identify places where additional support may be needed. For example, when surveys suggest older adults would like more time to practice activities in a session or seek further one-on-one tech time, an organizational decision can be made to increase the time of an individual session, create a variety of online materials, or develop a technical call hotline.

Conclusion: key programmatic and policy interventions

The practice guidelines presented in this case study can be used to inform policy as a multilayered approach to addressing digital inclusion. At the policy level, supports must be added to both debunk myths of technology adoption (such as older adults do not have interest in, or do not use, ICT) and guarantee resources are allocated to decrease barriers. Policies need to support programs that create technology acceptance through appropriate, age-based education and training, technology designed for the older learner, and for programs that offer broadband to older adults to increase connectivity (Davidson et al., 2012). Such policy interventions can continue the trend of increasing technology use among older adults.

Partnerships, policy change, and funding are needed to forward digital inclusion. Partnerships OATS cultivated are seen in Table 2. These partnerships are examples of how OATS worked with organizations to extend the reach of internet accessibility and programming to diverse groups of older adults. These partnerships ranged from OATS national connectivity consortium to get older adults online to working with older adults in NYC Public Housing to deliver empowering curriculum in English, Spanish, and Chinese. Collaborations resulted in the creation of materials dedicated to grandparents raising grandchildren and encountering new technology-based questions during the pandemic.

Policies need to support internet and broadband access specifically for older adults. These policies can follow changes made to telehealth access for older adults during the pandemic. The Health Information Technology for Economic and Clinical Health (HITECH) Act allowed for the expansion of technology use in healthcare delivery (Department of Health and Human Services, 2017). Through the supported policy expansion of telehealth (under Medicare, called Waiver 1135), some barriers to virtual visits were removed during COVID and may be extended beyond the pandemic. The waiver allows for full, paid coverage of telehealth visits outside of previous geographic restrictions and broadened the types of telehealth services provided (Centers for Medicare, 2020).

Other federal agencies have picked up on the theme of HITECH and Medicare's expansion of virtual healthcare provision. For example, the Administration for Community Living (ACL, 2021) along with the Centers for Medicare offered a webinar, "Bridging the Digital Divide for Home and Community Based Services Beneficiaries." The webinar recognized the impact of the digital divide in terms of access to services, health care, overall quality of life, and connectivity during the pandemic. It suggested:

> Many older adults and people with disabilities do not have the financial means to pay for internet service in their home nor purchase an internet enabled device - such as a PC, tablet, or smart phone. Further, many lack the skills needed to confidently navigate the internet and digital communities by themselves. This is particularly relevant with the transition to telemedicine and virtual services in place of in-person visits due to the COVID-19 public health emergency.

Though the call for decreasing the digital divide comes from a healthcare based or telehealth approach, the language of the legislation offers insight into how these policies can be used to decrease the gap between the "haves" and "have nots" and could play a meaningful role in reducing the digital divide. While the shift to digital learning was greatly accelerated by the COVID-19 pandemic, the guidelines suggested here for virtual programming that serves older adults have a broader applicability. Reducing barriers to virtual participation promotes older adults' full inclusion in the digital sphere.

ORCID

Joyce Weil (iD) http://orcid.org/0000-0002-1573-6534

References

Administration for Community Living. (2021 February 4). *Webinar: Bridging the digital divide for HCBS beneficiaries.* U.S. Department of Health & Human Services. https://acl.gov/nesws-and-events/announcements/aclcms-webinar-24-bridging-digital-divide-hcbs-beneficiaries

Armitage, R., & Nellums, L. B. (2020). COVID-19 and the consequences of isolating the elderly. *The Lancet*, (5), e 256. 5. https://doi.org/10.1016/S2468-2667(20)30061-X

Blaschke, C. M., Freddolino, P. P., & Mullen, E. E. (2009). Ageing and technology: A review of the research literature. *The British Journal of Social Work*, 39(4), 641–656. https://doi.org/10.1093/bjsw/bcp025

Centers for Medicare (2020 March 17) *Medicare telemedicine health care provider fact sheet.* U.S. Centers for Medicare & Medicaid Services. https://www.cms.gov/newsroom/fact-sheets/medicare-telemedicine-health-care-provider-fact-sheet

Charness, N., & Holley, P. (2004). The new media and older adults: Usable and useful? *American Behavioral Scientist, 48*(4), 416–433. https://doi.org/10.1177/0002764204270279

Chatterjee, P., & Yatnatti, S. K. (2020). Intergenerational digital engagement: A way to prevent social isolation during the COVID-19 crisis. *Journal of the American Geriatrics Society (JAGS), 68*(7), 1394–1395. https://doi.org/10.1111/jgs.16563

Davidson, C. M., Santorelli, M. J., & Kamber, T. (2012). Toward an inclusive measure of broadband adoption. *International Journal of Communication, 6*, 2555–2575.

Department of Health and Human Services (2017 June 16). *HITECH act enforcement interim final rule.* https://www.hhs.gov/hipaa/for-professionals/special-topics/hitech-act-enforcement-interim-final-rule/index.html

Estes, C. L. (2019). *Aging AZ: Concepts toward emancipatory gerontology.* Routledge.

Giorgi, M., & Ziegler, K. (2019a). *The OATS approach to curriculum design for senior planet programs.* OATS.

Giorgi, M., & Ziegler, K. (2019b). *Training methodology for senior planet programs.* OATS.

Glazebrook, A. H. (2020). *Technology acceptance and the interplay of social interdependence among a sample of urban older adults – An exploratory organizational case study* (doctoral dissertation), SUNY: Stony Brook, School of Social Welfare.

Glazebrook, A. H., & Sakow, M. 2020 August 10. *2020 mid-year program update.* Presentation. OATS.

Hou, J., Wu, Y., & Harrell, E. (2017). Reading on paper and screen among senior adults: Cognitive map and technophobia. *Frontiers in Psychology, 8*, 2225. https://doi.org/10.3389/fpsyg.2017.02225

Kamber, T. (2017). Fighting social isolation: A view from the trenches. *Public Policy & Aging Report, 27*(4), 149–151. https://doi.org/10.1093/ppar/prx027

Kamin, S. T., Lang, F. R., & Kamber, T. (2017). *"Social contexts of technology use in old age" (pp. 35-56). Gerontechnology: Research, practice, and principles in the field of technology and aging.* (Kwon, Ed). Springer Publishing Company.

Kwon, S. (Ed.). (2017). *Gerontechnology: Research.* practice, and principles in the field of technology and aging. Springer Publishing Company.

Lind, M., Bluck, S., & McAdams, D. P. (2020). More vulnerable? The life story approach highlights older people's potential for strength during the pandemic. *The Journals of Gerontology: Series B, 76*(2): e45–e48. *online first.* https://doi-org.unco.idm.oclc.org/10.1093/geronb/gbaa105

Losada-Baltar, A., Jiménez-Gonzalo, L., Gallego-Alberto, L., Pedroso-Chaparro, M. D. S., Fernandes-Pires, J., & Márquez-González, M. (2020). We're staying at home": Association of self-perceptions of aging, personal and family resources and loneliness with psychological distress during the lock-down period of COVID-19. *The Journals of Gerontology: Series B, 76* (2): e10-e16.. https://doi.org/10.1093/geronb/gbaa048.

National Telecommunication and Information Administration. (1994). *Falling through the net.* Census Bureau, Population Division. Education and Social Stratification Branch.

OATS. (2020). *Senior planet digital.* Older Adults Technology Services. Retrieved July 29, 2020. https://oats.org/world-class-programs/senior-planet-digital-2/).

OATS. (2021). *Indicators that matter.* Older Adults Technology Services. Retrieved March 29, 2021 at: https://oats.org/indicators-that-matter/

Pew Research Center. (2019). *Internet/broadband fact sheet.* https://www.pewresearch.org/internet/fact-sheet/internet-broadband/

Seifert, A., Cotten, S. R., & Xie, B. (2020). A double burden of exclusion? Digital and social exclusion of older adults in times of COVID-19. *The Journals of Gerontology: Series B, 76* (2020): e99–e103. online first.doi: 10.1093/geronb/gbaa098

Settersten, R. A., Jr., Bernardi, L., Härkönen, J., Antonucci, T. C., Dykstra, P. A., Heckhausen, J., Kuh, D., Mayer, K. U., Moen, P., Mortimer, J. T., Mulder, C. H., Smeeding, T. M., Van Der Lippe, T., Hagestad, G. O., Kohli, M., Levy, R., Schoon, I., & Thomson, E. (2020). Understanding the effects of Covid-19 through a life course lens. *Advances in Life Course Research, 45*, 100360. https://doi.org/https://doi.org/10.1016/j.alcr.2020.100360

Spears, J., & Zheng, R. (2020). Older adults' self-efficacy in computer use and the factors that impact their self-efficacy: A path analysis. *Educational Gerontology, 46*(12), 757–767. https://doi.org/10.1080/03601277.2020.1815976

Venkatesh, V., Morris, M. G., Davis, G. B., & Davis, F. D. (2003). User acceptance of information technology: Toward a unified view. *MIS Quarterly, 27*(3), 425–478. https://doi.org/10.2307/30036540

Weil, J. (2017). *Research design in aging and social gerontology: Quantitative, qualitative, and mixed methods.* Taylor & Francis.

Xie, B., Charness, N., Fingerman, K., Kaye, J., Kim, M. T., & Khurshid, A. (2020). When going digital becomes a necessity: Ensuring older adults' needs for information, services, and social inclusion during COVID-19. *Journal of Aging & Social Policy, 32*(1–11), 460–470. https://doi.org/10.1080/08959420.2020.1771237

Xiong, J., & Zuo, M. (2019). Older adults' learning motivations in massive open online courses. *Educational Gerontology, 45*(2), 82–93. https://doi.org/10.1080/03601277.2019.1581444

Yusif, S., Soar, J., & Hafeez-Baig, A. (2016). Older people, assistive technologies, and the barriers to adoption: A systematic review. *International Journal of Medical Informatics, 94*, 112–116. https://doi.org/10.1016/j.ijmedinf.2016.07.004

Ziegler, K., & Giorgi, M. (2019). *Teaching methodology for Senior Planet programs.* OATS.

Zubatsky, M., Berg-Weger, M., & Morley, J. (2020). Using telehealth groups to combat loneliness in older adults through COVID-19. *Journal of the American Geriatrics Society (JAGS), 68*(8), 1678–1679. https://doi.org/10.1111/jgs.16553

Concerns of Family Caregivers during COVID-19: The Concerns of Caregivers and the Surprising Silver Linings

Elizabeth Lightfoot, Rajean Moone, Kamal Suleiman, Jacob Otis, Heejung Yun, Courtney Kutzler and Kenneth Turck

ABSTRACT

COVID-19 has had an enormous impact on older people around the world. As family caregivers provide a good portion of the care for older people, their lives have been drastically altered by COVID-19 too. Our study is an in-depth exploration of the greatest concerns of family caregivers in the United States during COVID-19, as well as their perspectives on the benefits of caregiving during this global pandemic. We conducted in-depth interviews with a diverse sample of 52 family caregivers in the United States between May and September of 2020 over video conferencing using a semi-structured interview guide. Thematic analysis was conducted to ascertain our participants' perceptions. Caregiver's concerns were organized into six main themes, including social isolation, decline in mental health, decline in physical and cognitive functioning, keeping their family members safe from COVID-19, lack of caregiving support, and caregiving stress. The themes related to the benefits of caregiving during COVID-19 included: enjoyed the slower pace, increased time to spend together, deepened relationships, recognizing the resilience of family members, and caregiving innovations. Our in-depth study helps social workers understand the nature of caregiving stress during COVID-19, as well as the positive aspects of caregiving, even during a global pandemic.

The SARS-CoV-2 (COVID-19) global pandemic has had an enormous impact on older people and their family members. In the United States, roughly 80% of the 220,000 COVID-19 related deaths as of November 2020 have been people over the age of 65, with 32% of the deaths of people over age 85 (Centers for Disease Control, 2020). Aside from the flurry of medical research trying to understand the mechanics of COVID-19 and potential interventions to prevent or treat its devastating impacts, especially to older and immuno-compromised people, there is growing attention by scholars on how COVID-19 is affecting the psychological and social well-being of older people and their support systems. Much of the scholarly attention has focused on the psycho-logical and physical impacts of the social isolation older people are experien-cing because of physical distancing requirements (Berg-Weger & Schroepfer, 2020; Luchetti et al., 2020; Montgomery et al., 2020). There has been much less attention on the impacts of COVID-19 on the family caregivers of older people and people with disabilities, whose lives have also been dramatically altered. As family caregivers provide the bulk of care for older people and people with disabilities (AARP, 2020), this study focuses on COVID-19's impact on family caregivers of older people and people with disabilities, as well as family caregivers' perspectives of unexpected benefits of caregiving during this global pandemic.

In the United States, family caregivers are most often the primary caregivers to older people and adults with disabilities living in community settings (AARP, 2020). Even when their family members are living in long-term care settings, family members are important sources of care. Under normal cir-cumstances, family caregiving can be stressful, and numerous studies have found that family caregivers can experience negative consequences, such as increased health problems, increased levels of depression, and lower family income (Schulz & Eden, 2016). Conversely, other studies have highlighted the psychological and physical benefits of family caregiving, sometimes called caregiving gains or positive aspects of caregiving (Kramer, 1997; Roth et al., 2018). During the unprecedented changes to caregiving required under COVID-19, these stressors and perceived positive benefits to family caregiving could vary considerably.

While there has been a considerable amount of scholarly attention to family caregiving during this epidemic, so far this has mostly consisted of commen-taries or letters to the editor, pointing out various concerns about family caregiving during COVID-19 or giving advice for family caregivers and their support systems (Duong & Karlawish, 2020; Greenberg et al., 2020; Ickert et al., 2020; Killen et al., 2020; Lightfoot & Moone, 2020; Morley et al., 2020; Ruopp, 2020; Schlaudecker, 2020; Stokes & Patterson, 2020). Considering the unprecedented number of studies related to COVID-19 and general scholarly attention to the importance of family caregiving during COVID-19, there have been surprisingly few empirical studies that examine family caregivers during this pandemic (Savla et al., 2020). Those that exist include several explorations of the mental health of family caregivers during the early stages of COVID-19 using already existing panel studies. For example, both Park (2020), using the nationally representative Understanding America Study, and Gallagher and Wetherell (2020), using the United Kingdom's Understanding Society long-itudinal panel, found that family caregivers had higher levels of mental health problems during COVID-19 than non-caregivers. Likewise, two smaller stu-dies using locally collected survey data explored stress and concerns among family caregivers. Savla et al. (2020), using data from an April 2020 survey of

53 rural caregivers in Virginia, found that about two-thirds of caregivers were experiencing COVID-19 related stress and that those caregivers had limited caregiving supports and were more likely to experience role overload. Likewise, Cohen et al. (2020) conducted a survey in April 2020 of 80 Argentinian family caregivers of persons with dementia. They found that the most prominent concerns of Argentinian caregivers were not having paid help to assist with caregiving and fear of the spread of COVID-19. Altieri and Santangelo (2021) conducted a similar online survey in April of 84 Italian family caregivers of older adults with dementia and found that these caregivers were also experiencing high levels of stress, caregiver burden, and depression. While these studies help provide beginning evidence that COVID-19 is stressful for family caregivers, previous studies have not explored the nuances of family caregivers' concerns thus far, nor the perceived benefits of family caregiving.

Our study takes a qualitative approach to explore family caregiving during COVID-19, informed by the literature on caregiving strain and caregiving benefits or gains that is prominent in caregiving research. The literature on caregiving strains or burdens is extensive, typically relying on the Stress Process Model (Turner, 2009) which describes how increased caregiving responsibilities can be primary stressors for caregiving, and can cause role strains when new caregiving responsibilities alter the normal activities of the caregiver. During COVID-19, it seems obvious that increased responsibilities under COVID-19 as well as changed caregiving tasks could lead to even greater stress. Likewise, this study is also guided by the caregiving gain literature, which suggests that providing quality care can lead directly to caregiver benefits (Sanders, 2005). Our study, which draws on this strengths-based approach to understanding caregiving (Peacock et al., 2010), is an in-depth exploration of both the greatest concerns of family caregivers in the U.S. during COVID-19 as well as their perspectives on the benefits of caregiving during this global pandemic. The only other qualitative study we could find of family caregiving during COVID-19 was completed by Vaitheswaran et al. (2020) of family caregiving in India, which describes some concerns and needs of Indian family caregivers.

Our specific research questions are:

(1) What are the greatest concerns of family caregivers of adults over age 65 or adults with disabilities regarding family caregiving during the COVID-19 pandemic?
(2) What do family caregivers consider the benefits of caregiving of adults over age 65 or adults with disabilities during the COVID-19 pandemic?

Research design and methods

Design

This study used qualitative methods to explore complex phenomena of family caregiving during the COVID-19 pandemic. We collected data through semi-structured interviews with family caregivers, which allowed for rich narrative responses, and subsequent coded the data into themes. Our multi-ethnic research team included two faculty members, four graduate students, and one undergraduate student. All of our team members had older family members or other family members at-risk for COVID-19, including three that were caregivers of their older relatives, one that was living with their older relative, and others with their own health concerns. And, of course, all team members were personally affected by the COVID-19 restrictions. We talked regularly at team meetings about how our own experiences shaped our understanding of all aspects of this research project. Approval for the study was obtained through the University of Minnesota.

Sample

We recruited participants for this qualitative study through convenience sampling, primarily through e-mail and social media. We posted notices on a number of professional and other sites in Minnesota. In addition, we conducted outreach within our professional and personal networks and sent notices to nonprofit caregiver support providers to distribute study announcements to caregivers. Participants were not provided any incentives to participate. Most participants lived in Minnesota, with less than 20% of the participants living in other states. The average age of participants was 58, and the average age for the care recipients was 71. Of our participants, 65.5% were non-Hispanic whites, 11.5% were black, 11.5% were Asian American, and 9.6% were Latinx. Forty-six percent of care recipients lived in long-term care, 42% lived with their caregiver, and the rest lived in other community settings. Over 80% of the participants were female, and 43% of the caregivers said they were the only person caring for their loved ones. Among the 52 interviewees, 5 people were caring for two family members, and 46 people were caring for one family member, in total, 56 family members.

Instrument

We utilized a semi-structured interview guide. Semi-structured interviews allowed us to obtain similar information from all participants while allowing for additional probing (Kallio et al., 2016). The guide included 13 major questions, 15 corresponding probing questions, and 7 questions on demographics. We first asked participants a series of questions regarding the type of care they provided to their family members. Next, we asked them to discuss their three top concerns about caregiving during COVID-19. Later in the interview, we delved more deeply into these various concerns, including barriers to providing care. We also asked the caregivers to describe any benefits of caregiving during the COVID-19 pandemic. We pre-tested the interview guide with seven community members to ensure that the questions were clear and meaningful. The interview guide included contact information for programs and services for family caregivers to access after the interview.

Data collection

Data were collected through qualitative interviews lasting between 25 and 60 minutes from May to September 2020. Interviews were conducted in English (n = 37), Somali (n = 5), Spanish (n = 5), and Korean (n = 5) and recorded through a secure Zoom. The interviews conducted in Somali, Spanish and Korean were conducted by bilingual interviewers. Upon obtaining contact information, participants were assigned to a member of the research team who conducted the interview and completed the initial coding and a different member of the research team completing a coding check (see below for coding details). Each researcher contacted participants directly to schedule individual sessions based on participant and researcher availability. Following consent and the completion of interviews, video files were stored in a secured Box account accessible only to researchers.

Interviews in English were initially transcribed using Zoom's transcription feature and then each researcher reviewed the transcript and made necessary editing and proofreading corrections. Somali, Spanish, and Korean interviews were translated by the bilingual interviewer into an English transcript.

Data analysis

We conducted an inductive thematic analysis following the guidelines proposed by Braun and Clarke (2006) to explore themes related to the concerns and benefits of caregiving during COVID-19. We reviewed each transcript and assigned initial codes based on concepts that emerged from the narrative, regardless of where they occurred during the interview. Codes were noted in an Excel spreadsheet with corresponding quotes. Upon completion of the initial coding of all transcripts, researchers met to establish a final coding framework. Transcripts were independently verified using the coding framework by an additional member of the research team, resulting in each transcript being coded by two reviewers. The codes were then grouped into themes, with the research team distilling the descriptions of the themes. All the transcripts were reviewed a final third time by the first author to verify and clarify the established themes.

Limitations

This study had several limitations. First, there are obvious disadvantages to using a convenience sample, such as not being able to generalize the findings to other groups or a larger population. However, as this was an exploratory study aimed to gain an initial understanding of caregiving changes during a contemporary crisis, the sampling method seemed acceptable. Further, we did recruit broadly and obtained a sample that was diverse in age, race, and living situation. A related issue was that we used technology both to recruit participants (e-mail and social media) and to conduct the interviews. We were recruiting during the pandemic when many services were shut down, so we were not able to recruit directly at locations where we might have reached people with less access to technology. Thus, our sample only includes people who saw our recruitment materials. Of the people who indicated interest in participating in our project, we did not lose any participants because of our mode of technology, but we are not sure how many we did not reach initially. A final limitation to our study was that we had seven researchers conducting interviews and coding data. This could lead to differences in the nature of the interview, with different interviewer skills and behaviors leading to different participant responses. As suggested by Boutain and Hitti (2006), we trained interviewers, conducted practice interviews, and used a semi-structured interview guide to help moderate this limitation. Further, while we had multiple people code the data, all transcripts were coded three times, with the first author checking all coding for all transcripts.

Findings

We organized our findings into two categories of themes: concerns of caregivers during COVID-19 and benefits of caregiving during COVID-19. We found seven themes related to concerns of caregivers and five related to benefits of caregiving, which are laid out in Table 1. The following discusses the 12 themes, substantiated through participant quotes, as suggested by Sandelowski (1994) to help illustrate the themes.

Table 1. Major themes related to the concerns of caregivers and benefits of caregiving.

Concerns of Caregivers	Benefits of Caregiving
• Social Isolation of Family Member and Caregiver	• Enjoyed the Slower Pace
• Decline in Mental Health of Family Member	• Increased Time to Spend Together
• Decline in Physical & Cognitive Functioning of Family Member	• Deepened Relationships
	• Recognized the Resilience of their Family Members
• Keeping Family Members Safe from COVID-19	
• Lack of Caregiving Support	• Caregiving Innovations
• Caregiver Stress	

Concerns of caregivers during COVID-19

Our first category of themes focused on concerns caregivers had related to caregiving during COVID-19. Caregivers were asked directly about their greatest concerns at the beginning of the interviews and shared other concerns throughout their interviews. We identified seven themes of concerns of caregivers, including social isolation of the family member and caregiver, decline in the mental health of family members, decline in the physical and cognitive functioning of family members, keeping their family members safe during COVID-19, lack of caregiving support, and caregiver stress.

Social isolation of the family member and caregiver

The most common concern discussed by our participants was social isolation resulting from quarantining and physical distancing related to COVID-19. This theme was found in nearly every interview, and for several of our participants, was their only concern. Our participants discussed how COVID-19 had drastically limited their loved ones' social interactions, and how their own interactions had decreased substantially. For example, one caregiver providing care to her parents living in a retirement community said:

> I have teenagers . . . in the summers . . . when they didn't have school, they would go over there and have lunch with them four times a week to keep them company. But then now . . . . my parents haven't left their apartment. And no one has gone into their apartment.

Participants were concerned that the increased social isolation was causing their loved ones to feel sad, lonely, and bored, and expressed concern about how the isolation was affecting their loved ones' mental and physical health. For example, a caregiver who cares for her 75 year-old father living in an assisted living facility said that her greatest concern was "just the isolation, probably, like, the fact they're pretty much in their rooms . . . they can't do much else and just the impact isolation has on a person." While many of the caregivers were able to communicate with their loved ones by other means, a number described how both the caregivers and the care recipients miss being in the physical presence of each other. For example, a participant whose 89-year-old mother lives in memory care within an assisted living facility said, "I can't see her. I can't go visit her, I can stand outside or window and talk to her over the phone, but I can't get in to see her, which is huge." Similarly, a caregiver caring for her 81-year-old mother in her home detailed her mother's social isolation:

> Her family cannot even come to visit her, so her own children can't visit her. They just talk over the phone, because we are worried about the disease. Some of her siblings are around here, and they can't even come to her, so they talk to her on FaceTime sometimes. Because of that, she misses people.

While our participants were nearly universally worried about the effects of social isolation on their loved ones, the theme of social isolation also emerged as a concern about the caregivers themselves. Caregivers were intentionally isolating themselves because they needed to keep their loved ones safe. Caregivers expressed concern about how the social isolation was affecting their own well-being and ability to provide good care. For example, a 71-year-old caregiver caring for her partner in their home said, "I just can't have others be with me. So, I'm on a journey that is singular right now."

Participants were also concerned that social isolation would increase in the winter, when walks, outdoor activities, and some face-to-face visits from a distance would not be possible. For individuals suffering from cognitive impairments, virtual interactions can be too complex to navigate, leading many caregivers to feel anxious about how they will maintain connections during the winter. Additionally, aging individuals often rely on walks and outdoor activities for exercise, and will not be able to continue that when the weather becomes too cold. A participant who cares for her 81-year-old husband in a retirement community reflected:

> I keep saying I'm grateful that if this darned virus had to come now, that it came in the spring so we could be outdoors rather than it being February ... the weather has made such a difference, this would be a whole different can of worms if it were the winter.

Decline in mental health of family member

A common and related theme among our participants was the concern that social isolation was causing a decline in the mental health of their family members. The participants discussed declines in mental health—particularly depression and anxiety—as an acute result of social isolation. This was a prevalent concern of caregivers caring for family members living both in long-term care and community settings. For example, a caregiver of her 85-year-old father in an assisted living facility shared how her father was experiencing depression from being confined to a small, shared bedroom. She said, "He has enough awareness to where this is ... a source of anxiety and depression for him. And every time I talk to him he brings [his room] up."

The concern about the decline in mental health was slightly different for those who had dementia, as participants described the restrictions causing confusion and distress. For example, one caregiver described her 81-year-old mother, who was living with dementia within their shared home, as being distraught with her family, as she felt her family was responsible for the lockdown.

> That [social isolation] really affected her behavior, and her personality became more difficult. She sometimes feels that we are the ones doing this to her, and it's not happening to other people. She felt a lot of pressure, feeling that we are creating the pressure for her.

Decline in physical and cognitive functioning of family member

Another common theme of caregivers was their grave concern that that loved ones' physical and cognitive functioning would decline during the pandemic. They pointed to several factors that could cause these declines, notably social isolation, lack of opportunity to exercise, and lack of access to regular health care or therapies. Participants particularly pointed to social isolation as a cause of the declines in cognitive functioning of their loved ones, particularly among those living in facilities. While before COVID-19 they had plenty of activities to attend, opportunities for social interaction, and regular visits from family and friends, they now had little mental stimulation. Caregivers described their own efforts to provide mental stimulation for their loved ones, often from afar, but worried that these were not enough, particularly when their loved ones were no longer able to do independent activities, such as reading or watching television. Participants feared that this would lead to a cognitive decline in their loved ones, and many relayed how they could already see these declines.

Participants were also concerned that their loved ones were not getting the exercise they needed to maintain their physical health. Participants caring for relatives living in facilities and in the community discussed the canceling of regularly scheduled activities, such as exercise classes, as deleterious to their loved one's health. Some of those caring for family members in facilities worried that their loved ones were getting little exercise, both due to the canceling of activities and the lack of ability for family members to help their loved ones get exercise. For example, a caregiver of her 84-year-old mother in a facility said, "I don't think she's getting the exercise that she was getting before because they're not taking her."

Those providing care in the community also worried about their lack of ability to take their relatives out for exercise, as they did not want to expose their relative to COVID-19. For instance, a caregiver who lived with and cared for her 80-year-old mother relayed how she no longer felt safe to take her mother out for exercise: "We used to take her to walk around, to go to the mall, to get food, and now we can't do any of that. All day we just stay home."

Some participants discussed how they were worried that their loved ones' physical health would decline because they were no longer receiving regular health care or rehabilitation. Some discussed how medical appointments, elective surgeries, or physical therapy had been cancelled because of COVID-19. Others discussed being unable to take their family member to medical appointments for a variety of related reasons. Others described avoiding medical appointments as they feared they would not be able to physically accompany their loved one to an appointment, which was especially problematic if their family member did not speak English or had dementia. Finally, some avoided taking their family members to medical appointments as they were concerned that their family members would contract COVID-19 during the visit. For example, a caregiver providing care to both of her parents in their 70s in her home said:

> I worry about, like if they need to, they need health care. You know, and they take a lot of medicines and pills and, and I worry about what if I need to take them to the doctor. I just, I worry about their health.

Participants were also concerned that the COVID-19 restrictions would continue to be prolonged and the cognitive and physical declines would be so severe that their loved ones will not recover. For example, a woman caring for her 76-year-old father in a facility said she was concerned that he would decline so much that he would not be able to recover his functioning enough to enjoy meeting with his family members. She worried that, "by the time we end this COVID isolation, he would have gotten to the point where he can't look forward to those sorts of things." Similarly, another caregiver worried his 92-year-old mother would no longer recognize him, "I'm kind of fearful she's going to forget who I am without more regular contact than this."

Keeping family members safe from COVID-19

A common theme in our interviews was that caregivers were concerned about keeping their family members from contracting COVID-19. Every participant in our sample was caring for a relative with at least one risk factor for having severe COVID-19 symptoms, with many were caring for family members who had multiple risk factors. So, for many, one of their main concerns was keeping their loved ones safe. As put by a woman caring for her 97-year-old father living in a facility, her top concern was, "just, you know, wanting him to be safe from the virus." Participants expressed concern about how their relatives would fare if they contracted COVID-19, wondering not only if they would survive, but also how they would cope with the disease if they had to be hospitalized. For example, a caregiver caring for her 81-year-old mother in her home said:

> We worry that she will get the disease. If the person contracts the disease, you can't even go with them to the hospital and see them, you can't even sit with them to help them drink water. You can't stand next to your parent, and that creates a lot of worry for us.

Most caregivers prioritized safety as a major responsibility of caregiving and greatly altered their own lives to keep their relatives safe. A concern of many participants was that they would give their family member or another high-risk adult COVID-19. For example, a woman caring for her 76-year-old father in her home said, " . . . my biggest concern was what if I were the one to bring it home." Similarly, a woman caring for her 88-year-old mother in a memory care unit said, "I would just never forgive myself because of [the] asymptomatic nature of the virus if I walked in there and gave it to her . . . or if I gave it to somebody else." Caretakers also worried about their relatives contracting

COVID-19 from a staff member in a facility or from hired help in the home, and some had even terminated these services because of these concerns. For example, a caregiver of his 78-year-old mother at home said, "My other worry was that the disease will come into our apartment specifically because we used to have a lot of nurses coming to the apartment, so they could bring the disease inside."

Lack of caregiving support

Another theme emerging from our data was the participants' concerns about the lack of supports they had for caregiving. While the majority of our participants were not connected with formal caregiving supports, most had an informal support network. Many of those caring for relatives in their own home discussed forgoing formal or informal supports in their homes because of their concerns about COVID-19. Some related that before COVID-19 they shared responsibilities with other family members, but have since had to adjust their caregiving arrangements and redistribute the workload with some taking a larger share than before. Others discussed wanting to hire someone to help in the home but were unable to do it for financial reasons or concerns that hiring staff would increase the chance of COVID-19. For example, a woman caring for her 73-year-old husband in their home said, "I would really hesitate to have someone come in here because they might do more harm than good."

Caregiver stress

The final theme related to family caregiving that emerged was caregiver stress. These compounding themes created a cascading effect, with caregivers limiting their family member's interactions due to fear of COVID-19, resulting in social isolation of both the caregiver and care receiver and increased caregiving demands, which created worry about mental and physical well-being, all while working full-time from home in a house full of people. Others talked about how their own financial precarity, such as losing their own job or worrying about losing income because of COVID-19, exacerbated this stress. This stress was expressed by many participants. For example, a caregiver of her 73-year-old husband described the difficulties in providing care during COVID-19 as follows: "Just the emotional aspect of it that is so hard. You know, we, we love our person. And there, and there are times that we don't. It's just true. I mean, the truth is, it's hard to . . . It's hard to do."

Several talked about strategies to cope with the additional caregiving or as a 69-year-old woman caring for her 85-year-old husband put it, "Being able to maintain my own, um, you know, well-being and kindness." One participant described this as needing to put some emotional distance between her and her 98-year-old mother who lives in an assisted living facility, the big challenge on my part is staying emotionally, um, distant enough that I can support my mom without, I mean she is my mom, she reads when I'm upset, she reads when I'm sad. . . . So being able to support her and give her the strength and courage to say this is okay. It's not right, but it's okay.

Only a few participants talked directly about the need for self-care, with most of our participants more focused on the needs of their family members and competing concerns. One of the few who talked about self-care was a woman who cares for her elderly parents who live with her. She said,

You just kind of get sucked into all these places. And, you don't, take care of yourself. And I have a really great support system. I really do. But I just realized that it's really takes a toll on me that probably the effects, you know, other areas of my family and my life and how good I can be for myself and for others?

Benefits to caregiving during COVID-19

Our second category of themes focuses on benefits to caregiving during COVID-19. Most participants were able to identify at least one benefit of caregiving during COVID-19, however, four of our participants indicated that there were no positive aspects whatsoever to caregiving during the pandemic, and several more struggled to find anything positive. The five main themes related to benefits were enjoyed the slower pace, increased time to spend together, deepened relationships, recognized resilience in family members, and caregiving innovations.

Enjoyed the slower pace

The first theme that emerged as a benefit among all groups of participants was that participants enjoyed the slower pace of caregiving resulting from the COVID-19 related restrictions. Caregivers felt their lives had become less complicated. A woman who cared for her 85-year-old husband in her home said, "I'm not pulled in so many directions." The pandemic-related restrictions led caregivers to be able to focus more on caregiving and their own relationships. Caregiving during the pandemic became less of a chore, and with other distractions eliminated, they could pay closer attention to caregiving.

For some caregivers caring for relatives in long-term care settings, this slower pace resulted partially from not being able to visit their family member regularly. This barrier leads to conflicted feelings, as some caregivers felt guilty and worried about not providing care to their loved ones, yet at the same time were enjoying a less hectic schedule. As a woman caring for her 92-year-old mother in memory care said,

I'm more relaxed now ... where before I was constantly thinking ... I gotta arrange my schedule ... I think oddly enough, I probably am less stressed now in a way than I was before, because I can't see her, it's not even an issue.

Several also talked more generally about the slower pace of society, with fewer crowds and little traffic, which calmed both the caregivers and care recipients. Some participants talked about being able to take their loved ones out for exercise on quiet streets. Another said, "I could go grocery shopping without stress from cars and people."

While adapting to this new, slower paced schedule could be challenging, it was typically conceived as a temporary "break" from a hectic schedule, providing a needed respite for caregivers. However, this "break" was lasting too long for some people. For example, a woman caring for her 81-year-old husband in a retirement community-related, "So at least for the first month or two it was really kinda nice to have a break. Now it's getting old."

Increased time to spend together

Another strong theme relating to benefits for participants caring for family members in the community was the increased time they had to spend with each other. The safety precautions that caregivers were taking, along with local or state restrictions, resulted in family members spending much more time together with their loved ones. They described their families having time to play games, do puzzles, cook together, tell each other stories, and do other activities that they did not have time for before COVID-19. As one woman caring for her 72-year-old husband in the home said: "I spend more time with him. We have more one on one time where you know my focus is more on him and he thinks, and I do too, that we've gotten closer. And I don't know if that would have happened before."

This was especially the case for multigenerational families, with participants sharing how the lockdown had led to grandchildren spending much more time with their grandparent(s) living in their home. This was viewed as extremely beneficial for intergenerational family connections, and some viewed these benefits as enormous "gifts" for their families. The following sentiment by a woman caring for both her parents in her home was typical of this theme:

I mean it's just this time that we never would have had together. And I think we definitely see that is just a gift, you know, with my parents, the age that they are and my kids age that they are they, we never would have had this with, you know, the places we are in our life. So, it's really precious and it's a memory of time that we will always really treasure.

Deepened relationships

Perhaps the most common theme related to benefits was the deepened relationships amongst family members. These deepened relationships were especially strong for the participants who were caring for their family members in their own home. As COVID-19 had led people to a slower pace, some caregivers noticed a strengthening of family bonds. As one caregiver said about her husband she cares for, "He likes the time that we spend together. And also since I don't go outside that much, we are getting closer." Others talked about how this extended family time led them to get to know each other better. For example, a caregiver of her 81-year-old mother in her house said, "My mother tells them stories, they talk about different things, and they get to know each other."

Others described how their family relationships had deepened from caring for each other during the pandemic. A woman caring for her 75-year-old father in her home said she felt closer to her father as she noticed, "How we'll bend over backwards for each other to keep each other safe . . . I think you take [it] for granted." Similarly, another caregiver said she felt closer with her other family members as they all pitched in together to help her care for her parents, "I mean they've always been helpful, but to know that they're really there for me."

For those caring for relatives living in facilities or other locations outside their home, some described how they have also grown closer when limited to communicating over the phone or video. Some described how that while they were no longer visiting in person, they spent more time actually connecting to each other when communicating, which helped deepen their relationships. For example, a daughter caring for her 85-year-old father in a facility said,

> I think I was visiting him more and seeing him more . . . I was arranging family visits and I was taking him places so there wasn't as much talking. So, the silver lining is . . . we talked to him on the phone a lot and so we've heard a lot of stories. I've heard a lot of stories about when he was a kid and I've heard a lot of stories he was telling me, . . . and he was telling me stories about that and I'd never heard.

Others talked about how not being able to visit their family member in person led them to realize how important their family relationships are. For example, a caregiver caring for her 97-year-old father said, "I appreciated the ability to go into his apartment and see him or to have dinner with him. And maybe I just sort of took all that for granted before and now you know I do miss it."

Recognized the resilience of their family members

Another theme that emerged was that the COVID-19 restrictions resulted in them recognizing the resilience of their family members in ways they had not realized before. For family caregivers, their family member relying on them for doing certain tasks results in perceptions of dependency. This can lead some caregivers to worry about what would happen to their family members if they were not available to care for them. For some of our caregivers caring for family members living outside of the home, the COVID-19 restrictions which disallowed caregiver visits provided an opportunity to see how their family member would fare without them. For several caregivers in our study, they felt a sense of relief that their family members could cope without them. For example, this parent of an adult child with a disability highlighted a benefit of COVID-19:

> Seeing that [my daughter] has done as well as she has ... she's more adaptable than we thought she might be ... and thinking if she's getting through this, when the day comes, where she will need to live her life without us again.

Similarly, a caregiver to his 92-year-old mother woman in a facility humorously stated, "'I started thinking that if the apocalypse happens: cockroaches, Keith Richards, and my mom (will survive it).'"

Caregiving innovations

The final theme related to caregivers' perceived benefits of caregiving during COVID-19 were the innovations in caregiving. Participants particularly noted the innovative uses of existing technology for caregiving, such as video chatting, telehealth visits, virtual support opportunities, or home deliveries of groceries or prescriptions. While all the technologies that they mentioned were available before COVID-19, the restrictions related to COVID-19 led to the widespread adoption of these innovations by caregivers. These made their lives easier during the pandemic but also were generally helpful for caregiving. For example, participants used video chatting to connect with their loved ones during a quarantine or lockdown. However, after discovering that this worked well, they quickly expanded these video chats to include other family members living further away. While this technology had been available for years, many only first started connecting their loved ones with distant family members because of COVID-19. Telehealth was another innovation touted by caregivers, which was a good safety measure during COVID-19, but could also eliminate future driving to appointments, which is taxing on caregivers.

Discussion

The findings from this study illuminate both the concerns of family caregivers of caring during COVID-19 as well as the benefits of caregiving during the global pandemic. While several studies have pointed to the increased stress, caregiver burdens, and mental health challenges of family caregivers during COVID-19 (Park, 2020; Savla et al., 2020), our study helps to focus our understanding on the nature of this stress. Not surprisingly participants in our study described increased stress related to increased caregiving responsibilities during COVID-19 as well as a lack of adequate caregiving supports. These findings fit well with the traditional understanding of stress related to caregiving, including the Stress Process Model (Turner, 2009). For our participants, many of them did have increased caregiving responsibilities with inadequate supports, which caused increased stress, and this was acerbated with additional changes in caregivers' lives, such as working from home and/or homeschooling. Overall, the "normal" activities of caregiving were greatly altered under COVID-19, which the Stress Process Model suggests leads to increasing caregiver stress or strain.

The most pressing concerns for the majority of our participants, however, were their worries about the social isolation and health of their family members, as well as for their own health and well-being. Caregivers were concerned particularly about how the required social isolation of their loved ones, necessary to keep them safe, would lead to declines in the mental health and physical and cognitive functioning of their family members. While social isolation is a critical concern among gerontological social workers (Lubben et al., 2015), our family caregivers were mostly concerned about the outcomes of social isolation that was related to the physical isolation necessary because of the pandemic. While many caregivers tried to overcome these physical barriers through creative uses of technology, they were concerned with the lack of physical proximity to their loved one. Yet, at the same time, they also were greatly concerned about keeping their family members safe from COVID-19 itself, and greatly concerned about their family members getting sick or dying. These worries were fairly universal among our participants and these worries fit well with research on worries caregivers have when their family members were hospitalized (Li, 2005), though the contexts are different. Understanding the nuances of these competing stressors of caregiving during COVID-19 helps us understand why the panel and survey studies have shown higher mental health concerns among family caregivers during the pandemic (Gallagher & Wetherell, 2020; Park, 2020; Savla et al., 2020). In addition, it points to the need for social workers to develop and test more interventions for preventing social isolation and increasing family connections, including in situations where social isolation is necessitated for health or safety reasons. Further research could also examine the differences in caregiving stress during a crisis such as a pandemic based on culture, gender, age, relationship status, or other aspects.

Exploring caregiving during this unprecedented time allowed us to view the resiliency of caregivers and positive aspects of caregiving from a new light. There is a large body of literature that points to a variety of benefits, gains, or positive aspects of caregiving, such as feeling useful, feeling appreciated, fulfilling an obligation, strengthening relationships, learning of new skills, becoming more focused in the present and/or gaining a sense of strength (e.g., Koerner et al., 2009; Parveen & Morrison, 2012; Pendergrass et al., 2019; Roth et al., 2018). Numerous studies have also found that caregivers who viewed caregiving in a positive manner were more likely to have a higher perceived level of well-being (Quinn & Toms, 2019).

Our study differed from these typical studies, as our participants were focusing on the positive aspects of caregiving during a global pandemic, where their caregiving responsibilities often changed because of the pandemic-related restrictions. However, even under these difficult conditions, most participants could describe some positive aspects of caregiving during COVID-19. For those living with their loved ones, participants pointed primarily to how the restrictions to prevent the spread of COVID-19 had led them to have a slower paced life with more time to spend with their family members, which resulted in deepened, multi-generational relationships. Strengthened relationships are one of the benefits often discussed in the literature, though our participants described how the pandemic restrictions created much more opportunities for caregivers to spend more time with their family members, which was not always possible in their previous busy lives. This extended beyond the caregiving dyad, with participants also noting strengthened bonds between their older relatives and their grandchildren and extended family and friends. While we saw this as strong benefits for caregivers across cultures, a further culturally specific exploration would likely be even more illuminating.

For participants living apart from their family member, some also mentioned that they were able to deepen their connections, though this was typically through call or video chats, or their lack of ability to visit in person had led to a greater appreciation of their relationship. Some participants living apart also mentioned how the pandemic led them to better appreciate the resilience of their family members, learning that while their own caregiving role is important, their family members could function well without them too. Most caregivers also mentioned how the COVID-19 related restrictions had spurred the use of new technologies for caregiving and health care delivery, and some were using these technologies for many more connections than they had before. When the COVID-19 restrictions ease, social workers, and social work researchers can explore how some of these silver linings of caregiving during COVID-19 could be supported, and can also explore in more depth how the perceived benefits of caregiving during a crisis such as a pandemic varied across groups.

Conclusion

Those investigating or designing caregiver supports now and in the future could build upon these lessons learned about caregiving during COVID-19. Specifically, our knowledge of pandemic-specific stressors, such as the tandem legitimate worries about social isolation causing physical and mental health declines and the global worries about COVID-19, is an important avenue to address when developing plans for older adults and their family caregivers for times of crisis. Likewise, while strengthening family relationships are a well-known positive aspect of family caregiving, the severe COVID-19 restrictions amplified family caregivers' perceptions of this benefit. Thus, future plans for supporting family caregivers and their loved ones can build on this perceived benefit. Finally, this study's findings point to the importance of technology for increasing social connections or helping caregivers find ways to deepen their relationships, especially during crises that restrict physical connections. Overall, future research should target this adaptability and resilience of caregivers to further our understanding of caregiving during a crisis such as a global pandemic.

Funding

This work was supported by the Center for Healthy Aging and Innovation, University of Minnesota [N/A].

References

AARP. (2020, May). *Caregiving in the U.S.* American Association of Retired Persons. https://www.aarp.org/content/dam/aarp/ppi/2020/05/full-report-caregiving-in-the-united-states.doi.10.26419-2Fppi.00103.001.pdf

Altieri, M., & Santangelo, G. (2021). The psychological impact of COVID-19 pandemic and lockdown on caregivers of people with dementia. *The American Journal of Geriatric Psychiatry, 29*(1), 27-34. https://doi.org/10.1016/j.jagp.2020.10.009

Berg-Weger, M., & Schroepfer, T. (2020). COVID-19 pandemic: Workforce implications for gerontological social work. *Journal of Gerontological Social Work, 63*(6–7), 524–529. DOI:10.1080/01634372.2020.1772934

Boutain, D. M., & Hitti, J. (2006). Orienting multiple interviewers: The use of an interview orientation and standardized interview. *Qualitative Health Research, 16*(9), 1302–1309. https://doi.org/10.1177/1049732306290130

Braun, V., & Clarke, V. (2006). Using thematic analysis in psychology. *Qualitative Research in Psychology, 3*(2), 77–101. https://doi.org/10.1191/1478088706qp063oa

Centers for Disease Control. (2020, November 1). *CDC COVID data tracker.* https://covid.cdc.gov/covid-data-tracker/

Cohen, G., Russo, M. J., Campos, J. A., & Allegri, R. F. (2020). Living with dementia: Increased level of caregiver stress in times of COVID-19. *International Psychogeriatrics, 32*(11), 1377–1381. doi:10.1017/S1041610220001593

Duong, M. T., & Karlawish, J. (2020). Caregiving at a physical distance: Initial thoughts for COVID-19 and beyond. *Journal of the American Geriatrics Society, 68*(6), 1170–1172. https://doi.org/10.1111/jgs.16495

Gallagher, S., & Wetherell, M. A. (2020). Risk of depression in family caregivers: Unintended consequence of COVID-19. *BJPsych Open, 6*(6), 1–5. https://doi.org/10.1192/bjo.2020.99

Greenberg, N. E., Wallick, A., & Brown, L. M. (2020). Impact of COVID-19 pandemic restrictions on community-dwelling caregivers and persons with dementia. *Psychological Trauma: Theory, Research, Practice, and Policy, 12*(S1), S220. https://doi.org/10.1037/tra0000793

Ickert, C., Rozak, H., Masek, J., Eigner, K., & Schaefer, S. (2020). COVID19: Maintaining resident social connections during COVID-19: Considerations for long-term care. *Gerontology and Geriatric Medicine, 6*, 2333721420962669. https://doi.org/10.1177/2333721420962669

Kallio, H., Pietilä, A.-M., Johnson, M., & Kangasniemi Docent, M. (2016). Systematic methodological review: Developing a framework for a qualitative semi-structured interview guide. *Journal of Advanced Nursing, 72*(12), 2954–2965. https://doi.org/10.1111/jan.13031

Killen, A., Olsen, K., McKeith, I. G., Thomas, A. J., O'Brien, J. T., Donaghy, P., & Taylor, J. P. (2020). The challenges of COVID-19 for people with dementia with Lewy bodies and family caregivers. *International Journal of Geriatric Psychiatry, 35*(12), 1431–1436. https://doi.org/10.1002/gps.5393

Koerner, S. S., Kenyon, D. B., & Shirai, Y. (2009). Caregiving for elder relatives: Which caregivers experience personal benefits/gains? *Archives of Gerontology and Geriatrics, 48*(2), 238–245. https://doi.org/10.1016/j.archger.2008.01.015

Kramer, B. J. (1997). Gain in the caregiving experience: Where are we? What next? *The Gerontologist, 37*(2), 218–232. https://doi.org/10.1093/geront/37.2.218

Li, H. (2005). Hospitalized elders and family caregivers: A typology of family worry. *Journal of Clinical Nursing, 14*(1), 3–8. https://doi.org/10.1111/j.1365-2702.2004.01013.x

Lightfoot, E., & Moone, R. P. (2020). Caregiving in times of uncertainty: Helping adult children of aging parents find support during the COVID-19 outbreak. *Journal of Gerontological Social Work, 63*(6–7), 542–552. DOI: 10.1080/01634372.2020.1769793

Lubben, J., Gironda, M., Sabbath, E., Kong, J., & Johnson, C. (2015). Social isolation presents a grand challenge for social work. Grand Challenges for Social Work Initiative, Working Paper No, 7.

Luchetti, M., Lee, J. H., Aschwanden, D., Sesker, A., Strickhouser, J. E., Terracciano, A., & Sutin, A. R. (2020). The trajectory of loneliness in response to COVID-19. *American Psychologist, 75*(7), 897–908. https://doi.org/10.1037/amp0000690

Montgomery, A., Slocum, S., & Stanik, C. (2020, October). *Experience of nursing home residents during the pandemic: What we learned from residents about life under COVID-19 restrictions and what we can do about it.* Ann Arbor, MI: Altarum. https://altarum.org/sites/default/files/uploaded-publication-files/Nursing-Home-Resident-Survey_Altarum-Special-Report_FINAL.pdf

Morley, G., Sese, D., Rajendram, P., & Horsburgh, C. C. (2020). Addressing caregiver moral distress during the COVID-19 pandemic. *Cleveland Clinic Journal of Medicine.* Advance online publication. https://doi.org/10.3949/ccjm.87a.ccc047

Park, S. S. (2020). Caregivers' mental health and somatic symptoms during COVID-19. *The Journals of Gerontology: Series B.* Advance online publication. https://doi.org/10.1093/geronb/gbaa121

Parveen, S., & Morrison, V. (2012). Predicting caregiver gains: A longitudinal study. *British Journal of Health Psychology, 17*(4), 711–723. https://doi.org/10.1111/j.2044-8287.2012.02067.x

Peacock, S., Forbes, D., Markle-Reid, M., Hawranik, P., Morgan, D., Jansen, L., Leipert, B. D., & Henderson, S. R. (2010). The positive aspects of the caregiving journey with dementia: Using a strengths-based perspective to reveal opportunities. *Journal of Applied Gerontology, 29*(5), 640–659. https://doi.org/10.1177/0733464809341471

Pendergrass, A., Mittelman, M., Graessel, E., Özbe, D., & Karg, N. (2019). Predictors of the personal benefits and positive aspects of informal caregiving. *Aging & Mental Health, 23*(11), 1533–1538. https://doi.org/10.1080/13607863.2018.1501662

Quinn, C., & Toms, G. (2019). Influence of positive aspects of dementia caregiving on caregivers' well-being: A systematic review. *The Gerontologist*, *59*(5), e584–e596. https://doi.org/10.1093/geront/gny168

Roth, D. L., Brown, S. L., Rhodes, J. D., & Haley, W. E. (2018). Reduced mortality rates among caregivers: Does family caregiving provide a stress-buffering effect? *Psychology and Aging*, *33* (4), 619. https://doi.org/10.1037/pag0000224

Ruopp, M. D. (2020). Overcoming the challenge of family separation from nursing home residents during COVID-19. *Journal of the American Medical Directors Association*, *21*(7), 984–985. https://doi.org/10.1016/j.jamda.2020.05.022

Sandelowski, M. (1994). Focus on qualitative methods. The use of quotes in qualitative research. *Research in Nursing & Health*, *17*(6), 479–482. https://doi.org/10.1002/nur.4770170611

Sanders, S. (2005). Is the glass half empty or half full? Reflections on strain and gain in caregivers of individuals with Alzheimer's disease. *Social Work in Health Care*, *40*(3), 57–73. https://doi.org/10.1300/J010v40n03_04

Savla, J., Roberto, K. A., Blieszner, R., McCann, B. R., Hoyt, E., & Knight, A. L. (2020). Dementia caregiving during the "stay-at-home" phase of COVID-19 pandemic. *The Journals of Gerontology Series B: Psychological Sciences and Social Sciences*. Advance online publication. https://doi.org/10.1093/geronb/gbaa129

Schlaudecker, J. D. (2020). Essential family caregivers in long-term care during the COVID-19 pandemic. *Journal of the American Medical Directors Association*, *21*(7), 983. https://doi.org/10.1016/j.jamda.2020.05.027

Schulz, R., & Eden, J. (Eds.). (2016). *Families caring for an aging America*. National Academies Press.

Stokes, J. E., & Patterson, S. E. (2020). Intergenerational relationships, family caregiving policy, and COVID-19 in the United States. *Journal of Aging & Social Policy*, *32*(4–5), 416–424, DOI:10.1080/08959420.2020.1770031

Turner, R. J. (2009). Understanding health disparities: The promise of the stress process model. In Avison, W.R., Aneshensel, C.S., Schieman, S., Wheaton, B. (Eds.), *Advances in the conceptualization of the stress process: Essays in Honor of Leonard I. Pearlin* (pp. 3–21). Springer.

Vaitheswaran, S., Lakshminarayanan, M., Ramanujam, V., Sargunan, S., & Venkatesan, S. (2020). Experiences and needs of caregivers of persons with dementia in India during the COVID-19 pandemic—A qualitative study. *The American Journal of Geriatric Psychiatry*, *28* (11), 1185-1194. https://doi.org/10.1016/j.jagp.2020.06.026

Is It "Aging" or Immunosenescence? The COVID-19 Biopsychosocial Risk Factors Aggravating Immunosenescence as Another Risk Factor of the Morbus. A Developmental-clinical Social Work Perspective

Robert K. Chigangaidze(iD) and Patience Chinyenze(iD)

ABSTRACT

COVID-19 has proliferated ageism. The impetus of this article is to show that immunosenescence is a risk factor to COVID-19 and not aging per se. Based on the idea that some older people are also healthier than younger ones, the emphasis of this article is on immunosenescence and not aging as a risk factor of COVID-19 complications. The paper utilizes a biopsychosocial approach to expound on the link between immunosenescence and COVID-19 risk factors. The article explores biological factors such as malnutrition, comorbidities, substance abuse, and sex. It also expands on psychosocial factors such as mental health disorders, homelessness, unemployment, lack of physical exercises, stigma, and discrimination. The article calls for gerontological social work to assume a developmental-clinical social work perspective to prevent the early onset and progression of immunosenescence. It calls for gerontological social work to prevent factors that promote unhealthy aging. The article promotes a preventative stance to practice and not just curative approaches. Treatment involves primary prevention which emphasizes on avoiding the onset of unhealthy aging. It is this approach that gerontological social work should aim also to address in building resilience in the face of pandemics.

The risks of developing severe complications from COVID-19 and dying from it increase with age (Wu & McGoogan, 2020; Sciacqua et al., 2020). Deaths per million from COVID-19 rise dramatically with age, increasing from 23.6, 66.6, and 159.1 respectively among individuals aged 33–44, 45–54, and 55–64 years, to 377.9 and 969.8 among individuals aged 65–74 and 75–84 years and an astonishing 2,670.6 for individuals 85 years and older (Miller, 2020, p. 299). In the initial phase of the pandemic, death rates were 11.4 times higher among those 80[+] than they were for people aged 50–59 years (Reher et al., 2020:2). A large proportion of COVID-19 deaths occurred in long-term care facilities that care for the elderly with physical and cognitive impairments in need of assistance with basic activities of daily living such as eating, bathing and toileting (Miller, 2020). The main question that this article seeks to address is whether it is aging or immunosenescence that is putting people at risk of COVID-19 complications.

During the COVID-19 pandemic we face an exacerbation of ageism (Meisner, 2020; Previtali et al., 2020). COVID-19 has also exposed socio-economic inequalities that are present in welfare systems, health services, and other human organizations (Henrickson, 2020; Krouse, 2020). The pandemic is also exacerbating these socio-economic inequalities that aggravate immunosenescence and weaken people's resilience in the face of health adversities. COVID-19 has exposed both the resiliency of the elderly population and the challenge to ensure that this large and diverse population can access the resources, information and services they need (Morrow-Howell et al., 2020). Social determinants such as poverty, high crime neighborhoods, poor access to healthy foods, limited education and skill level, and high unemployment increase the risk of chronic diseases and infection from COVID-19 (Krouse, 2020; Reeves & Rothwell, 2020). If these social determinants are not addressed, there will be an early onset and progress on immunosenescence.

Immunosenescence is a canopy term that is used to describe age-related declines in the normal functioning of the immune system (Bigley et al., 2013). "Aging" is accompanied by the remodeling of the immune system which leads to a decline in the immune efficacy over time (Aiello et al., 2019). Immunosenescence predisposes the elderly to increased risks of heart diseases, respiratory infections, pneumonia, and various noncommunicable diseases (NCDs) (Bencivenga et al., 2020; Gavazzi & Krause, 2002; Pawelec, 2018). Aging can be associated with immunosenescence which aggravates the likelihood for COVID-19 complications (Calder, 2020). The fulcrum of our argument is that aging is not the sole pathway to immunosenescence. Several factors such as genetics, nutrition, exercise, previous exposure to infections, sex and gender, and human cytomegalovirus (HCMV) status can influence immunosenescence (Aiello et al., 2019; Maijó et al., 2014; Xu et al., 2020). As we explore on this concept, it is important to appreciate that the global community is undergoing a substantial shift in demographics. The number of individuals aged more than 60 years is increasing dramatically (Weinberger, 2016).

Negative age stereotyping is currently taking place on a devastating scale in light with COVID-19. Proclamations that elderly people are uniformly categorized as "at risk" pose great psychosocial harm to them (Ehni & Wahl, 2020). Elderly patients are now being deemed disposable when it comes to treatment triaging and countries like Italy, Spain, Brazil, United Kingdom, and some states in the United States of America have experienced these devastating effects (Lichtenstein, 2020). Utilizing the clinical perspective of the biopsychosocial approach and the developmental perspectives of the critical theory, anti-oppressive theory, and ecological systems thinking, we seek to expose some social inequalities that affect the elderly. This disquisition supports the claim that "aging" is not a risk factor as some elderly people are also healthier than younger ones. We advance the need to integrate both the developmental and clinical social work perspectives in enhancing the welfare of the elderly, whereas research proposes that targeting the aging process itself can be a viable orthogonal strategy against COVID-19 (Santesmasses et al., 2020), we put forward an argument that interventions should target immunosenescence not aging. We advise that if the biopsychosocial factors aggravating immunosenescence were addressed over the course of life, this would enhance resilience to the COVID-19.

First and foremost, we will outline our assumptions for the purposes of our argument. The discussion on how COVID-19 affects the immune system will follow. The article will conceptualize the developmental-clinical social work perspective and biopsychosocial approach to COVID-19. Thereafter, it will explore on the biopsychosocial risk factors of COVID-19. The article will also illustrate that the same risk factors of COVID-19 also aggravate immunosenescence. To its end, it will call for social workers to adopt a developmental-clinical social work approach that builds on resilience and prevents an early onset of immunosenescence.

Assumptions

1. The elderly people are at remarkably high risk of adverse outcomes from COVID-19 infections because of decreased immune competence [immunosenescence] (Cox et al., 2020; Cunha et al., 2020; Napoli et al., 2020).
2. Immunosenescence can start in childhood due to viral infections (Dalzini et al., 2020).
3. Immunosenescence is influenced by biopsychosocial factors (Aiello et al., 2019).
4. Addressing the causes of immunosenescence can contribute to better resilience and lessen the morbus burden in the face of health ppandemics, such as COVID-19 in future.

COVID-19 and the immune system

COVID-19 activates the innate immune system resulting in the release of large numbers of cytokines causing cytokine storms, which are associated with multiple organ failure. The cytokine storm accounts for acute respiratory distress syndrome and is the cause of most COVID-19 related deaths (Hojyo et al., 2020). A cytokine storm has also been found in people receiving chemotherapy, in diabetes patients and other chronic conditions (Erener, 2020; Filippou & Karagiannis, 2020). The cytokine storm reflects an immune system that has gone wrong. Immunosenescence is characterized by a reduced ability to mount an adequate immune response to adversity and the predisposition of the proinflammatory state, such as cytokine storm (Nidadovulu & Walston, 2020). Put simply, the dysregulation of the immune system is often referred to as immunosenescence. An immune system that has gone malfunctional. Research can also explore how COVID-19 can reduce viral resilience in people who recover from its severe complications (Mueller et al., 2020).

The developmental-clinical social work perspective

Grounded in the thinking of Van Breda (2018) of the developmental social casework, this paper seeks to expand the concept of developmental social work to clinical social work practice. For the purposes of this article, developmental-clinical social work is the integration of social development concepts and those of clinical social work to prevent the prevalence of disease, minimize its burden, and builds on community resilience. Developmental-clinical social work also reflects on the biological, psychological and socio-economic inequalities that affect disease prevalence in the life course of the population.

This article integrates the aspects of critical social work, ecological systems theory, anti-oppressive theory, structuralism, functionalism, and a human rights perspective into clinical social work. Critical social work distinguishes the past and present, mostly characterized by domination, exploitation, and oppression, and a possible future rid of these issues (Granter, 2009). Critical social work and the anti-oppressive theory are embedded in the emancipation of humanity from structural oppression. The paper will look on the biological, psychological, and social issues from a structural way and appreciate that a person's welfare is affected by the micro, meso, exo, macro and chronosystems (Chigangaidze, 2020). Human rights are fundamental in health issues because the latter is inherent of the former. There are no human rights without the focus of health. Human rights are inclusive of the highest attainable health, prevention of diseases, optimum housing, adequate water, and sanitation, food and nutrition. It is in this background that we advance the developmental-clinical social work perspective in Gerontological Social Work.

The impetus of the developmental-clinical social work perspective is to prevent human suffering by means of tracing the pathways through which diseases are aggravated. It articulates that prevention is better than cure. It emphasizes on resilience and a strength-based perspective to the prevention of diseases. The developmental-clinical social work perspective advances for the minimization of disease burden. Thus, it is concerned with the reduction of the morbidity and mortality rates of the morbus through addressing biopsychosocial factors aggravating the morbus.

Conceptualizing the biopsychosocial approach to COVID-19

The Biopsychosocial Approach (Engel, 1977) is a multimodal and interdisciplinary model that explores the interactional relationship between the biological, psychological and socio-environmental influences on health and diseases (Frazier, 2020). This model is utilized in clinical social work and other fields (Harkness, 2011). The biopsychosocial approach to health and disease emphasizes that illness is beyond the biomedical model but rather includes the state of the organism with equally important biological, psychological and social factors (Havelka et al., 2008 as cited in Chigangaidze, 2020). The Biopsychosocial Approach relates to the person-in-the-environment perspective of social work practice. It emphasizes that the person does not exist in a vacuum. However, the biopsychosocial approach is limited in that it fails to account for the spiritual component to human behavior and phenomenon. Whereas the biopsychosocial approach has been extended to the spiritual domain (Katerndahl, 2008; Sulmasy, 2002), we will only expound on the biological, psychological and social factors for the sake of space and time. The spiritual domain will be considered in a distinct paper.

Biological factors

The following section will explore on malnutrition, substance abuse, comorbidities and sex. These factors are risk factors to COVID-19 and aggravate immunosenescence which is greatly increasing the disease burden of COVID-19 among the elderly. We have put forward an illustration as Figure 1 for the benefit of explaining our argument.

Malnutrition

Malnutrition in all its forms has become the leading cause of ill health and death, and the rapid rise of diet-related NCDs in straining the health systems (Development Initiatives, 2020). Malnutrition is prevalent among approximately one-third of the elderly, especially in those with institutionalized facilities (Sciacqua et al., 2020). Malnutrition in the early ages of life has been implicated in the development of NCDs in later ages of life (World Health Organization, 2014) contributing to weakening of the immune system. This aggravates one's predisposition to developing complications when infected with COVID-19 (Chigangaidze, 2020). Malnutrition is a major geriatric syndrome due to multifaceted etiology, characterized by muscle wasting and weight loss, which is strongly related to frailty and negative outcomes (Bencivenga et al., 2020). COVID-19 has also affected the access to food by the elderly due to lockdowns (Cohen & Tavares, 2020; Miller, 2020).

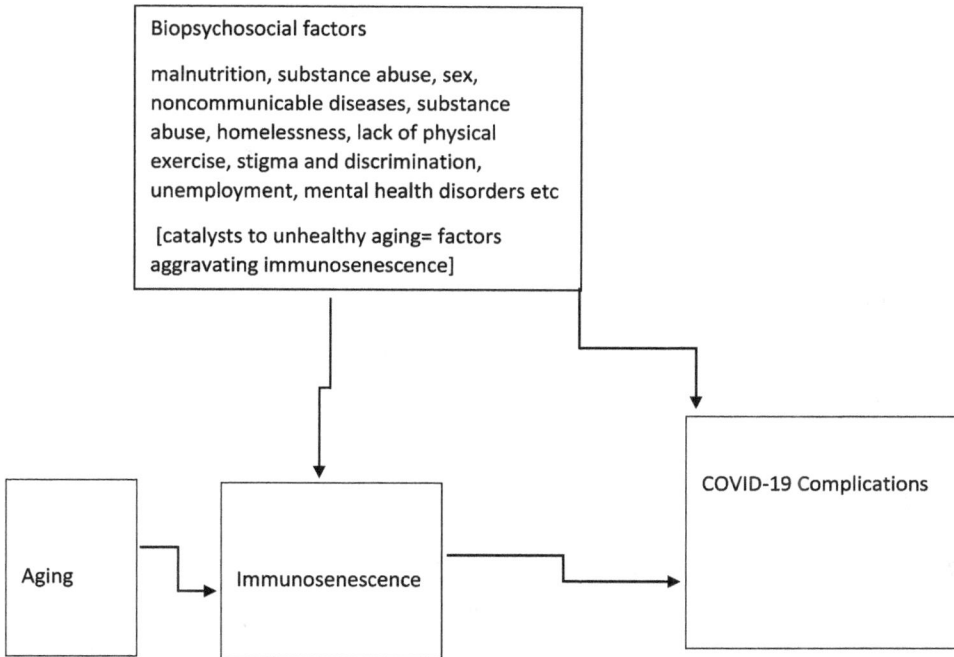

Figure 1. Notes:Biopsychosocial factors aggravating immunosenescence are the same that are associated with COVID-19 complications.If immunosenescence can occur in childhood, then it would be injustice to say aging is its sole contributor. The Biopsychosocial factors can contribute to immunosenescence as both individual factors or as co-existing factors.

Social workers are involved in food security issues and enhance the access to such basic needs to vulnerable members of the community, including the elderly. Social work should advocate for better access to adequate and nutritious food by all people as this helps in building resilience by means of slowing the onset of immunosenescence. Nutrition has the capacity to unveil the biological outcomes of inequalities and discriminatory practices (Eide, 2002). Social work practice in gerontology and other domains is engraved in advancing human rights. Social work should take the lead in the fight against hunger as food insecurity poses great threats to contemporary human security and the early onset as well as progress of immunosenescence.

Substance abuse

The abuse of substances is also identified as a risk of developing COVID-19 related complications (Kong et al., 2020). Substances such as methamphetamine, cocaine, alcohol and marijuana have been implicated in the early onset of immunosenescence and its progression (Zaparte et al., 2019; Potula et al., 2018). Substance abuse, especially alcohol abuse, contributes to malnutrition as it has been implicated in the inhibition of optimum absorption of nutrients, such as Vitamin B-1 (Thiamine) resulting in Korsakoff syndrome leading to an early onset and progression of immunosenescence (Bunout, 1999; Lieber, 2003, 1995; Rossi et al., 2015). Substance abuse has also been implicated as one factor contributing to the rise of noncommunicable diseases associated with COVID-19 complications and immunosenescence (Chigangaidze, 2020; Comer, 2013). The role of social work is to enhance interventions targeting the primary treatment (prevention) of substance abuse and intervening at all stages of the ecological systems with the aim of reducing the burden of substance abuse thereby building on resilience in the face of health adversities.

Comorbidities

Comorbidities in the form of NCDs, such as cancer, hypertension, diabetes mellitus, cardiovascular problems, and others, as well as communicable diseases have also been associated with COVID-19 complications (Mills, 2020; Rahimi & Abadi, 2020; United Nations, 2020). Noncommunicable diseases are inextricably linked to natural aging processes (Yiengprugsawan & Browning, 2019). The World Health Organization reports that NCDs were responsible for 40.5 million or 71% of the global deaths in 2016 (Allen & Feigl, 2017). It is essential to state that these statistics have already exceeded the projections of the World Health Organization that by 2030 noncommunicable diseases will account for about 70% of the deaths (Hunter & Reddy, 2013). As stated before in this paper, deprivations to adequate nutrition predispose one to risks of suffering from noncommunicable diseases in the later stages of life. It is essential that clinical social workers, developmental clinical social workers, and "developmental-clinical social workers" advocate for the prioritization of food security at all times as this goes a long way in the prevention of noncommunicable diseases, thereby enhancing community resilience in times of adversity such as pandemics.

We argue in this section that interventions targeting immunosenescence begin at the prenatal stage or even earlier than that. Fetal alcoholic spectrum disorders (FASDs) that result from substance abuse during pregnancy are also associated with the development of noncommunicable diseases that weaken the immune system at the later ages of life. Thus, counseling techniques such as motivational interviewing and efforts to stop substance abuse by pregnant women can go a long way in the fight against comorbidities implicated in COVID-19 complications as well as immunosenescence. Genetic testing and counseling have also proven to play an important critical life-saving role for family members, such as in the case of colon cancer (Jamaluddine et al., 2016). Other interventions to reduce the prevalence of immunosenescence and the factors associated with COVID-19 complications by means of preventing the occurrence of comorbidities will be discussed in the next sections.

Gender

Men's COVID-19 related mortality rates are higher than that of women (Bentron et al., 2020). Research to answer why more males are dying than women is increasing. In a recent study, scientists collected plasma samples of 331 patients who were COVID-19 positive and women were found to be containing more antibodies compared to men (Biswas, 2020 as cited in Chigangaidze, 2020). The biopsychosocial nature of being male or female contributes to gender disparities of lifespan and longevity. We appreciate that:

> Women live longer than men and this difference in life expectancy is a worldwide phenomenon indicating that human longevity seems strongly influenced by gender defined as the combination between biological sexual characteristics (anatomy, reproductive functions, sex hormones, expression of genes on X or Y chromosome) and factors related to behavior, social role, lifestyle and life experiences. (Ostan et al., 2016, p. 1711)

Thus, even in longevity males are also disadvantaged due to both natural causes and behavioral issues. In relation to COVID-19, the virus has shown to be disproportionately affecting males compared to females in terms of mortality rates. It is important that social workers consider addressing issues that relate to behavioral change among men, for example, enhancing health seeking behaviors, such as stopping substance abuse without also sidelining females.

Psychosocial factors

This section will explore the lack of physical exercise, mental health disorders, homelessness, unemployment, stigma and discrimination in relation to COVID-19 and immunosenescence.

Lack of physical exercises

Sedentary lifestyle increases risks of major noncommunicable diseases and is fourth on the list of the leading causes of death worldwide (Oloo et al., 2017). It is well documented that regular participation in moderate-intensity exercise attenuates age-related oxidative stress and reduces the frequency of several immune biomarkers that are associated with compromised immunity. This implies that exercise may delay the onset of immunosenescence and attenuate the risk of infection including COVID-19 (Azizi et al., 2020). Physical activity has been identified as one of the effective ways in the prevention and treatment of noncommunicable diseases that also pose risks of developing COVID-19 complications (McKenzie, 2012). It has been emphasized that physical exercises are not only beneficial for the prevention and treatment of some non-communicable diseases but also delays the onset and progress of immunosenescence. Thus, it is necessary for practitioners in gerontology to schedule time for physical exercises for the elderly in collaboration with other members of the multidisciplinary team. We appreciate the excellent work done by the 100 years old Captain Tom Moore who even raised funds for the National Health Services through physical exercises.

Mental health disorders

People with mental health problems are at an increased rate for COVID-19 infection (Yao et al., 2020). The proliferation of COVID-19 has led to the increase of anxiety as people become worried about their lives and survival (Thakur & Jain, 2020). Late-life depression and anxiety are diseases that aggressively affect health and shorten the immunity (Rybka et al., 2009). Anxiety is a kind of psychological stress that presents with a series of physiological events and it can cause a decline in immunity (Liu et al., 2020; World Health Organization, 2020). The elderly are predisposed to these mental disorders especially at the lockdown periods because of social loneliness. The messages advancing ageism may also increase the levels of anxiety among the elderly population. Social workers need to encourage the elderly to engage in meditation and yoga as these may improve physical and mental health (Shibani, 2013). There is need to prevent the occurrences of mental health disorders during an individual's life course to reduce the burden associated with these disorders in late stages of life. This is also intertwined with interventions targeting the homeless, substance abuse, food iinsecurity, and unemployment to enhance one's psychosocial functioning.

Homelessness

Homeless populations are more prone to low immunity and to lack of public hygiene, inadequate waste disposal, and poor-quality mental health predisposing them to COVID-19 complications (Barnejee & Bhattacharya, 2020; Krouse, 2020). It is well documented that older homeless persons suffer from substantially more physical illness than their non-homeless peers (Cohen, 1999). Compared to the general elderly population, elderly homeless people are in worse health, have higher mortality rates and tend to die at a younger age . Homelessness tends to increase the rate of immunosenescence, thereby aggravating the chances of COVID-19 infection. Thus, both developmental social workers and clinical social workers should enhance housing projects and programs to mitigate disease burden secondary to immunosenescence related to homelessness. There are also socio-structural factors that lead to homelessness among the elderly and these include poverty, poor housing schemes, and unemployment (Mayock & Sheridan, 2012). We advise that social workers in gerontology may address these socio-structural issues to lessen the prevalence of homelessness among the elderly, thereby delaying the onset of immunosenescence.

Unemployment

Unemployment decreases the functionality of immune function (Burgard et al., 2007; Cohen et al., 2007). People who are unemployed are more at risk to COVID-19 hospitalizations also because of socio-economic inequalities (Bambra et al., 2020). Unemployment reduces one's health insurances and even access to health facilities for regular checks thereby making early diagnosis and treatment of chronic diseases difficult resulting in early onset and progression of immunosenescence. Unemployment reduces one's access to nutritious food, better housing, and a healthy lifestyle which impacts negatively on the immune system thereby exposing one to early onset and progression of immunosenescence. Unemployment can be associated with reduced physical activity and promotes a sedentary lifestyle which catalyzes immunosenescence. Thus, gerontological social workers may consider being involved in advocacy against the rising unemployment rates of youths as this greatly affects their workload in the future as evidenced that unemployment promotes unhealthy aging. Interventions to reduce unhealthy aging may adopt a social change approach to address unemployment since it has been implicated in the early onset of immunosenescence.

Stigma and discrimination

Stigma has been explored as leading to the development of negative attitudes toward the elderly such as ageism, prejudices, damaging self-beliefs, discrimination in the provision of services for physical health problems (Holm et al., 2014). In this pandemic, there are reports of triaging systems that have placed the elderly at low priority in the treatment of COVID-19 (D'cruz & Banerjee, 2020). Discrimination as a determinant of health and wellbeing can promote unintended or intended unhealthy behaviors (Jackson et al., 2019). Social media is a useful tool for health promotion but during the pandemic it has been negatively used to express antagonistic stereotypes, prejudice and discrimination against the elderly (Meisner, 2020). Stigma and discrimination have severe effects on biopsychosocial functioning of anyone as it makes one vulnerable even to suicidal ideation, substance abuse, stress disorders, and other mental health problems. Stigma and discrimination limits early diagnosis and treatment of diseases among the aging, thereby negatively impacting on their recovery.

Implications

Social work in gerontology should aim at preventing unhealthy aging as a pathway to reduce the burden of pandemics such as COVID-19 in future. Preventing the onset and progression of immunosenescence is key as it builds on resilience and immune competence in the face of health adversities. We argue in this paper for a paradigm shift in gerontological social work. We advise that social work practice in gerontology should assume a preventative approach to unhealthy aging and not just settle for the remedial interventions. We put forward the need for social workers to adopt a developmental-clinical social work perspective to fight biopsychosocial factors that exacerbate immunosenescence. Social work needs to be an agent of social change and not an instrument of social control. It must face the socio-structural issues contributing to the early onset and progression of immunosenescence head-on. COVID-19 is a call for social workers in gerontology to rethink of their professional mandate and offer helpful interventions in the form of preventing the prevalence of unhealthy aging. In doing so, social work acknowledges that pandemics are fought before they emerge by means of establishing resilience and delaying the onset of immunosenescence. A developmental-clinical social work perspective will address ageism and deal with the biopsychosocial aspects that contribute to immunosenescence. Treatment involves primary prevention which emphasizes on avoiding the onset of unhealthy aging. It is this approach that gerontological social work should aim also to address in building resilience in the face of pandemics. We question in this paper if immunosenescence is age-related and if aging is a risk factor to COVID-19.

Conclusion

The article has shown that "aging" is not the main factor contributing to COVID-19 complications but immunosenescence. It has emphasized that gerontological social work can adopt a developmental-clinical social work perspective which is preventative of unhealthy aging, early onset, and progression of immunosenescence. The paper has called for social workers to address the biopsychosocial factors aggravating the early onset and progression of immunosenescence. We argue that COVID-19 is a call for a preventative stance in gerontological social work practice. Is aging a curse? Have we not proliferated ageism? The world could seek alternatives of making a milieu that addresses immunosenescence for the betterment of life in the elderly ages. We have argued that pandemics are fought before they emerge through ensuring resilience and healthy aging. Fellow colleagues let us refrain from "ageism"." Let the love for diversity and humanity lead. Above all, let us leave a legacy of hope, love and humanness (ubuntu) to generations to come. It could be injustice and limiting to say aging is a risk factor to COVID-19.

ORCID

Robert K. Chigangaidze ⓘ http://orcid.org/0000-0002-3597-8776
Patience Chinyenze ⓘ http://orcid.org/0000-0002-7341-9473

References

Aiello, A., Farzaneh, F., Candore, G., Caruso, C., Davinelli, S., Gambino, C. M., Ligotti, M. E., Zareian, N., & Accardi, G. (2019). Immunosenescence and its hallmarks: How to oppose aging strategically? A review of potential options for therapeutic intervention. *Frontiers in Immunology*, *10*(2247), 1–19. https://doi.org/10.3389/fimmu.2019.02247

Allen, L. N., & Feigl, A. B. (2017). Reframing non-communicable diseases as socially transmitted Conditions. *The Lancet Global Health*, *5*(7), e644–6. https://doi.org/10.1016/S2214-109X(17)30200-0

Azizi, G. G., Orsini, M., Júnior, S. D. D., Viera, P. C., De Carvalho, R. S., Pires, C.-S. D.-S., Cardoso, C. E., Mareno, A. M., & Azizi, M. A. A. (2020). COVID-19 and physical exercise: What is the relation between exercise immunology and the current pandemic situation? *Revista Brasileira De Fisiologia Do Exercício*, *19*(2Supl), S20–S29. https://doi.org/10.33233/rbfe.x19:2.4115

Bambra, C., Riordan, R., Ford, J., & Matthews, F. (2020). The COVID-19 pandemic and health inequalities. *Journal of Epidemiology and Community Health*, *74*, 964-968. jech-2020-214401. https://doi.org/10.1136/jech-2020-214401

Banerjee, D., & Bhattacharya, P. (2020). The hidden vulnerability of homelessness in the COVID-19 pandemic: Perspectives from India. International Journal of Social Psychiatry, 1–4. doi:10.1177/0020764020922890

Barker, R. L. (2003). *The Social Work Dictionary* (Fifth ed.). National Association of Social Workers.

Bencivenga, L., Rengo, G., & Varricchi, G. (2020). Elderly at the time of Coronavirus disease 2019 (COVID-19): Possible role of immunosenescence and malnutrition. *GeroScience*, *42* (4), 1089–1092. https://doi.org/10.1007/s11357-020-00218-9

Bentron, M., Gottert, A., Pulerwitz, J., Shattuck, D., & Stevanovic-Fenn, N. (2020). Men and COVID-19: Adding a gender lens. Global Public Health, 15 (7), 1090–1092. https://doi.org/10.1080/17441692.2020

Bigley, A. B., Spielmann, G., LaVoy, E. C. P., & Simpson, R. J. (2013). Can exercise-related improvements in immunity influence cancer prevention and prognosis in the elderly? *Maturitas*, *76*(1), 51–56. https://doi.org/10.1016/j.maturitas.2013.06.010

Biswas, R. (2020). Are men more vulnerable to COVID-19 as compared to women? *Biomedical Journal of Scientific & Technical Research*, *27*(2), 20645–20646. https://doi.org/10.26717/BJSTR.2020.27.004481

Bunout, D. (1999). Nutritional and metabolic effects of alcoholism: Their relationship with alcoholic liver disease. *Nutrition*, *15*(7–8), 583. https://doi.org/10.1016/S0899-9007(99)00090-8

Burgard, S. A., Brand, J. E., & House, J. S. (2007). Toward a Better Estimation of the Effect of Job Loss on Health. *Journal of Health and Social Behavior*, *48*(4), 369–384. https://doi.org/10.1177/002214650704800403

Calder, P.C. (2020). Nutrition, immunity and COVID-19. BMJ Nutrition, Prevention & Health. doi:10.1136/bmjnph-2020-000085

Chigangaidze, R. K. (2020). Risk factors and effects of the morbus: COVID-19 through the biopsychosocial model and ecological systems approach to social work practice. *Social Work in Public Health*, *36*(2), 98–117. https://doi.org/10.1080/1918.2020.1859035

Cohen, C. I. (1999). Aging and homelessness. *The Gerontological Society of America*, *39* (1),5–14. https://doi.org/10.1093/geront/39.1.5

Cohen, F., Kemeny, M. E., Zegans, L. S., Johnson, P., Kearney, K. A., & Stites, D. P. (2007). Immunede clines with unemployment and recovers after stressor termination. *Psychosomatic Medicine*, *69*(3), 225–234. https://doi.org/10.1097/PSY.0b013e31803139a6

Cohen, M. A., & Tavares, J. (2020). Who are the most at-risk older adults in the COVID-19 Era? It's not just those in nursing homes. *Journal of Aging & Social Policy*, *32*(4–5), 380–386. https://doi.org/10.1080/08959420.2020.1764310

Comer, R. J. (2013). *Abnormal Psychology* (Eighth ed.). Worth Publishers.

Cox, L. S., Bellantuono, I., Lord, J. M., Sapey, E., Mannick, J. B., Partridge, L., Gordon, A. L., Steves, C. J., & Witham, M. D. (2020). Tackling immunosenescence to improve COVID-19 outcomes and vaccine response in older adults. *The Lancet*, *1*(2), e55- e57. https://doi.org/10.1016/S2666-7568(20)30011-8

Cunha, L. L., Perazzio, S. F., Azizi, J., Cravedi, P., & Riella, L. V. (2020). Remodelling of the immune system with Aging: Immunosenescence and its potential impact on COVID-19 immune response. *Frontiers in Immunology*, *11*(1748), 1–11. https://doi.org/10.2289/fimmu.2020.01748

D'cruz, M., & Banerjee, D. (2020). 'An invisible human rights crisis: The marginalization of older during the COVID-19 pandemic – An advocacy review. *Psychiatry Research*, *292*, 113369. https://doi.org/10.1016/j.psychres.2020.113369

Dalzini, A., Petrara, M. R., Ballin, G., Zanchetta, M., Giaquinto, C., & De Rossi, A. (2020). Biological aging and immune senescence in children with perinatally acquired HIV. *Journal of Immunology Research*, *2020*, 1–15. Article ID 8041616. https://doi.org/10.1155/2020/8041616

Development Initiatives. (2020). *2020 Global Nutrition Report: Action on equity to end malnutriion.*

Ehni, H.-J., & Wahl, H.-J. (2020). Six prepositions against ageism in the COVID-19 pandemic. *Journal of Aging & Social Policy*, *32*(4–5), 515–525. https://doi.org/10.1080/08959420.2020.1770032

Eide, W. B. (2002). Nutrition and human rights. In *Nutrition: A foundation for development*. ACC/SCN.

Engel, G., . L. (1977). The need for a new medical model: A challenge for biomedicine. *Science*, *196*(4286), 535–554. https://doi.org/10.1126/science.847460

Erener, S. (2020). Diabetes, infection risk and COVID-19. *Molecular Metabolism*, *39*(101044), 1–10. https://doi.org/10.1016/j.molmet.2020.101044

Filippou, P. S., & Karagiannis, G. S. (2020). Cytokine storm during chemotherapy: A new companion diagnostics emerges? *Oncotarget*, *11*(3), 213–215. https://doi.org/10.18632/oncotarget.27442

Frazier, L. D. (2020). The past, present and future of the biopsychosocial model: A review of the biopsychosocial model of health and disease: New philosophical and scientific developments by Derek Bolton and Grant Gillet. *New Ideals in Psychology*, *57*(100755). https://doi.org/10.1016/j.newideapsych.2019.100755

Gavazzi, G., & Krause, K.-H. (2002). Ageing and infection. *The Lancet Infectious Diseases*, *2* (11), 659–666. https://doi.org/10.1016/S1473-3099(02)00437-1

Granter, E. (2009). Critical Social Theory and the End of Work. (1st Edition). London: Routledge

Harkness, D. (2011). The diagnosis of mental disorders in clinical social work: A review of standa rds of care. *Clinical Social Work Journal*, 39(3–4), 330–338. https://doi.org/10.1007/s10615-010-0263-8

Havelka, M., Lucanin, J. D., & Lucanin, D. (2008). Biopsychosocial model-the integrated approach to health and disease. *CollegiumAnthropologicum*, 33(1), 303–310.

Henrickson, M. (2020). Kiwis and COVID-19 : The Aote aroa New Zealand response to the global pandemic. The International Journal of Community and Social Development, 2 (2), 121-133. https:doi.org/10.1177/2516602620932558

Hojyo, S., Uchida, M., Tanaka, K., Hasebe, R., Tanaka, Y., Murakami, M., & Hirano, T. (2020). How COVID-19 induces cytokine storm with high mortality. *Inflammation and Regeneration*, 40(37), 1–7. https://doi.org/10.1186/s41232-020-00146-3

Holm, A. L., Lyberg, A., & Severinsson, E. (2014). Living with stigma: Depressed elderly person's experiences of physical health problems. *Nursing Research and Practice*, 2014, 1–8. https://doi.org/10.155/2014/527920

Hunter, D. J., & Reddy, K. S. (2013). Non communicable diseases. *The New England Journal of Medicine*, 369(14), 1336–1343. https://doi.org/10.1056/NEJMra1109345

Jackson, S. E., Hackett, R. A., & Steptoe, A. (2019). Associations between age discrimination and health and wellbeing: Cross-sectional and prospective analysis of the English long-itudinal study of ageing. *The Lancet Public Health*, 4(4), 200–208. https://doi.org/10.1016/S2468-2667(19)30035-0

Jamaluddine, Z., Sibai, A. M., Othman, S., & Yazbek, S. (2016). Mapping genetic research in non-communicable disease publications in selected Arab countries: First step towards a guided research agenda. *Health Research Policy and Systems*, 14(81). https://doi.org/10.1186/s1296-0153-9

Katerndahl, D. A. (2008). Impact of spiritual symptoms and their interactions on health services and life satisfaction. *The Annals of Family Medicine*, 6(5), 412–420. https://doi.org/10.1370/afm.886

Kong, K. L., Chu, S., & Giles, M. L. (2020). Factors influencing the uptake of influenza vaccine vary among different groups in the hard-to- reach population. *Australian and New Zealand Journal of Public Health*, 44(2), 163–168. https://doi.org/10.1111/1753-6405.12964

Krouse, H. J. (2020). COVID-19 and the widening gap in health inequality. *Otolaryngology - head and Neck Surgery*, 163(1), 65–66. https://doi.org/10.1177/0194599820926463

Lichtenstein, B. (2020). From "coffin dodger" to "boomer remover": Outbreaks of Ageism in three countries with divergent approaches to Coronavirus Control. *Journals of Gerontology Social Sciences*, 76(4), 1–7. https://doi.org/10.1093/geronb/gbaa102

Lieber, C. S. (1995). Medical disorders of alcoholism. *The New England Journal of Medicine*, 333(16), 1058–1065. https://doi.org/10.1056/NEJM199510193331607

Lieber, C. S. (2003). Relationships between nutrition, alcohol use and liver disease. *Alcohol Research & Health*, 27(3), 220–231.

Liu, K., Chen, Y., Wu, D., Lin, R., Wang, Z., & Pan, L. (2020). Effects of progressive muscle relaxation on anxiety and sleep quality in patients with COVID-19. *Complementary Therapies in Clinical Practice*, 39, 101132. https://doi.org/10.1016/j.ctcp.2020.10.1132

Maijó, M., Clements, S. J., Ivory, K., Nicoletti, C., & Carding, S. R. (2014). Nutrition, diet and immunosenescence. Mechanisms of Ageing and Development, 136–137, 116–128. https://doi.org/10.1016/j.mad.2013.12.003

Mayock, P., & Sheridan, S. (2012). Women's Journeys' to homelessness: Key findings from a biographical study of homeless women in Ireland. Research Paper 1. Dublin: School of Social Work and Social Policy and Children's Research Centre, Trinity College Dublin

McKenzie, D. C. (2012). Respiratory physiology: Adaptations to high –level exercise. *British Journal of Sports Medicine*, 46(6), 381. https://doi.org/10.1136/bjsports-2011-090824

Meisner, B. A. (2020). Are you OK, Boomer? Intensification of ageism and intergenerational tensi- ons on social media amid COVID-19. *Leisure Sciences*, *42*(5–6), 482–501. https://doi. org/10.1080/01490400.2020.1773983

Miller, E. A. (2020). Protecting and improving the lives of older adults in the COVID-19 Era. *Journal of Aging and Social Policy*, *32*(4–5), 297–309. https://doi.org/10.1080/08959420.2020. 1780104

Mills, S. (2020). COVID-19, public health measures, legal considerations: A medical perspective. *Judicial Review*,*25*(2), 71-79 . https://doi.org/10.1080/10854681.2020.1760575

Morrow-Howell, N., Galucia, N., & Swinford, E. (2020). Recovering from the COVID-19 pandem ic : A focus on older adults. *Journal of Aging & Social Policy*, *32*(4–5), 526–535. https://doi.org/10.1080/08959420.2020.1759758

Mueller, A. L., McNamara, M. S., & Sinclair, D. A. (2020). Why does COVID-19 disappropri- ately affect older people? *Aging*, *12*(10), 9959–9981. https://doi.org/10.18632/aging.103344

Napoli, C., Tritto, I., Mansueto, G., & Ambrosio, G. (2020). Immunosenescence exacerbates the COVID-19. *Archives of Gerontology and Geriatrics*, *90*(104174), 104174. https://doi.org/10. 1016/j.archger.2020.104174

Nidadovulu, L. S., & Walston, J. D. (2020). Underlying vulnerabilities to the cytokine storm and adverse COVID-19 outcomes in the Aging Immune System. *The Journals of Gerontology: Series A*, *76*(3), e13- e18. glaa2009. https://doi.org/10.1093/gerona/glaa209

Oloo, M. O., Kweyu, I., & Sabiri, E. (2017). Exercise and chronic diseases. International Journal of Science and Research (IJSR), 6 (10), 6–391. doi:10.21275/ART20177057

Ostan, R., Monti, D., Gueresi, P., Bussolotto, M., Franceschi, C., & Baggio, G. (2016). Gender, agi ng and longevity in humans: An update of an intriguing /neglected scenario paving the way to a gender-specific medicine. *Clinical Science*, *130*(19), 1711–1725. https://doi.org/10. 1042/cs20160004

Pawelec, G. (2018). Age and immunity: What is "immunosenescence"? *Experimental Gerontology*, *105*, 4–9. https://doi.org/10.1016/j.exger.2017.10.024

Potula, R., Haldar, B., Cenna, J. M., Sriram, U., & Fan, S. (2018). Methamphetamine alters T cell cycle entry and progression: Role in immune dysfunction. *Cell Death Discovery*, *4*(44). https://doi.org/10.1038/s41420-018-0045–6

Previtali, F., Allen, L. D., & Varlamova, M. (2020). Not only virus spread: The diffusion of ageism during the outbreak of COVID-19. *Journal of Aging & Social Policy*, *32*(4–5), 506–514. https://doi.org/10.1080/08959420.2020.1772002

Rahimi, F., & Abadi, A. T. B. (2020). Practical strategies against the novel coronavirus and COVID-19 – The imminent global threat. *Archives of Medical Research*, *51*(3), 280–281. https://doi.org/10.1016/j.jhin.2020.03.017

Reeves, R., & Rothwell, J. (2020). *Class and COVID: How the Less Affluent Face Double Risks*. Brookings Institution.

Reher, D., Requena, M., De Saints, G., Esteve, A., Bacci, M.L., Padyab, M., & Sandstrom, G. (2020). The COVID-19 pandemic in an aging world. doi:10.31235/osf.io/bfvxt

Rossi, R. E., Conte, D., & Massironi, S. (2015). Diagnosis and treatment of nutritional deficiencies in alcoholic liver disease: Overview of available evidence and open issues. *Digestive and Liver Disease*, *47*(10), 819–825. https://doi.org/10.1016/j.dld.2015.05.021

Rybka, J., Kedziora-Kornatowska, K., Kedziora, J., & Kucharski, R. (2009). Immunosenescence and late life depression. *CentralEuropean Journal of Immunology*, *34*(4), 271–275.

Santesmasses, D., Castro, J. P., Zenin, A. A., Shindyapina, A. V., Gerashchenko, M. V., & Gladyshev, V. N. (2020). COVID-19 is an emergent disease of aging. *GERO Aging Therapeutics Project*. https://doi.org/10.1101/2020.04.15.20060095

Sciacqua, A., Pujia, R., Arturi, F., Hribal, M. L., & Montalcini, T. (2020). COVID-19 and elderly: Beyond the respiratory Drama. *Internal and Emergency Medicine, 15*(5), 907–909. https://doi.org/10.1007/s11739-020-024-x

Shibani, N. (2013). *"Immunosenescence and exercise-mediated modulation of the innate immune response to influenza in mice."* Graduate Thesis and Dissertations, 13342. https://lib.dr.iastate.edu/etd/13342.

Sulmasy, D. P. A. (2002). Biopsychosocial-spiritual model for the care of patients at the end of life. *The Gerontologist, 42*(suppl_3), 24–33. https://doi.org/10.1093/geront/42.suppl_3.24

Thakur, V., & Jain, A. (2020). COVID 2019-suicides: A global psychological pandemic. *Brain, Behavior, and Immunity, 88*, 952–953. https://doi.org/10.1016/j.bbi.2020.04.062

United Nations. (2020). *COVID-19 and human rights: We are all in this together.*

Van Breda, A. (2018). Developmental social case work: A process model. *International Social Work, 61*(1), 66–78. https://doi.org/10.1177/0020815603783

Weinberger, B. (2016). Immunosenescence: The importance of considering age in health and disease. *Clinical and Experimental Immunology, 187*(1), 1–3. https://doi.org/10.1111/cei.12879

World Health Organization. (2014). *Global nutrition targets 2025: Stunting policy brief.* Retrieved August 2, 2020, from. www.who.int/nutrition/publications/globaltargets2025_policybrief_stuting/en

World Health Organization. (2020). *Addressing human rights as key to the COVID-19 response.*

Wu, Z., & McGoogan, J.M. (2020). Characteristics of and important lessons from the Coronavirus disease 2019(COVID-19) outbreak in China: Summary of a report of 72 314 cases from the Chinese Center for Disease Control and Prevention. JAMA, 323 (13):1239–1242. doi:10.1001/jama.2020.2648

Xu, W., Wong, G., Hwang, X. Y., & Larbi, A. (2020). The untwining of immunosenescence and aging. *Seminars in Immunopathology, 42*(5), 559–572. https://doi.org/10.1007/s00281-020-00824-x

Yao, H., Chen, J.-H., & Xu, Y.-F. (2020). Patients with mental health disorders in the COVID-19 epidemic. *The Lancet Psychiatry, 7*(4), 7. https://doi.org/10.1016/S2215-0366(20)30090-0

Yiengprugsawan, V. S., & Browning, C. J. (2019). Non communicable diseases and cognitive impairment: Pathways and shared behavioral risk factors among older Chinese. *Fontiers in Public Health, 7*(296). https://doi.org/10.3389/fpubh.2019.00296

Zaparte, A., Schuch, J. B., Viola, T. W., Baptista, T. A. S., Beidacki, A. S., Do Prado, C. H., Sanvicente- Viera, B., Bauer, M. E., & Grassi-Oliveira, R. (2019). Cocaine use disorder is associated with changes in Th1/ Th2, Th17 cytokines and lymphocytes subsets. *Fontiers in Immunology, 10*(2435). https://doi.org/10.3389/fimmu.2019.02435

Index

For Product Safety Concerns and Information please contact our EU
representative GPSR@taylorandfrancis.com
Taylor & Francis Verlag GmbH, Kaufingerstraße 24, 80331 München, Germany